Outpatient Case Management

Strategies for a New Reality

Edited by
Michelle Regan Donovan
and Theodore A. Matson

AHA books are published by
American Hospital Publishing, Inc.,
an American Hospital Association company

Library of Congress Cataloging-in-Publication Data

Outpatient case management : strategies for a new reality / edited by
  Michelle Regan Donovan, Theodore A. Matson.
     p.   cm.
  Includes bibliographical references.
  ISBN 1-55648-119-5 (pbk.)
  1. Ambulatory medical care—United States. 2. Hospitals—Case
management services. 3. Health care reform—United States.
I. Donovan, Michelle Regan. II. Matson, Theodore A.
  [DNLM: 1. Ambulatory Care—organization & administration—United
States. 2. Delivery of Health Care—trends—United States. WX 205
0938 1994]
RA974.084 1994
362.1'0973—dc20
DNLM/DLC
for Library of Congress   94-9597
                                                    CIP

Catalog no. 027100

Printed in the USA

Text set in English Times
3M—06/94—0372

Audrey Kaufman, Acquisitions and Development Editor
Nancy Charpentier, Production Editor
Peggy DuMais, Production Coordinator
Cheryl Kusek, Cover Designer
Marcia Bottoms, Books Division Assistant Director
Brian Schenk, Books Division Director

Contents

Part I

Part II

List of Figures

List of Tables

About the Editors

Michelle Regan Donovan, BSN, RN, is a principal with Ambulatory Care Advisory Group, Inc., in Chicago. A graduate of Georgetown University, she has more than 20 years' health care experience in the clinical, operational, and administrative realms of outpatient care. She lectures and writes frequently on topics related to outpatient and emergency care, focusing on strategies to enhance service delivery and contain costs. Ms. Donovan serves as advisor to various national committees, groups, and organizations on topics related to emergency, ambulatory and home care, facility design, and industry-focused environmental trends.

Theodore A. Matson, MA, CHE, is president of Ambulatory Care Advisory Group, Inc., a Chicago-based firm providing professional advisory, consultation, and management services exclusively for ambulatory care and emergency services. Previously, he was a manager with the Division of Ambulatory Care and Society for Ambulatory Care Professionals of the American Hospital Association, also in Chicago. Mr. Matson is a national and international speaker on ambulatory care, and frequently writes about ambulatory care topics. He is coauthor and editor of several texts, including *The Hospital Emergency Department: Returning to Financial Viability* (1986), *Restructuring for Ambulatory Care: A Guide to Reorganization* (1990), *Information Systems for Ambulatory Care* (1990), and *The Hospital Emergency Department: A Guide to Operational Excellence* (1992), all published by American Hospital Publishing, Inc. He currently is editor of "Outpatient Care," a column devoted to outpatient technologies in the monthly journal *Administrative Radiology*. A graduate of the University of Iowa, Mr. Matson is a member of both the Society for Ambulatory Care Professionals and a diplomate of the American College of Healthcare Executives.

Contributors

Joel E. Abrams, MSW, is a clinical social worker with the AIDS Services Diagnostic Evaluation Unit of the Johns Hopkins University School of Medicine's Division of Infectious Diseases, in Baltimore. He has provided diverse services to clients with HIV infection for seven years at Johns Hopkins and HERO, a community-based, private, not-for-profit organization.

Patricia Alario, RN, MS, CANP, is the manager of the Employee Health/Occupational Health Clinic at Burbank Hospital in Fitchburg, Massachusetts. Ms. Alario previously held various clinical and administrative positions for OMNI Health Systems in Natick, Massachusetts. She is currently a member of the Legislative Committee for the Central Mass Association of Occupational Health Nurses. Ms. Alario was a contributing author to *The Corporate Heart: Guidelines to Cardiovascular Health Promotion Programs in Business and Industry,* published by the American Heart Association.

Lawrence H. Bernstein, MD, is assistant clinical professor of medicine at the University of Connecticut School of Medicine, in Storrs. Dr. Bernstein serves on the board of directors of the Visiting Nurse Association of America and the American Academy of Home Care Physicians. Previously, he has been on the Joint Commission on Accreditation of Healthcare Organizations' Home Care Accreditation Committee. Currently, Dr. Bernstein is in private practice in Storrs, Connecticut, and is a consultant to the home care industry.

Mary Jo Breslin, RN, BSN, is an independent surgical services consultant. Previously, she was administrative director of surgical services at Georgetown University Hospital in Washington, DC. She is an active member of the American Organization of Nurse Executives and the Association of Operating Room Nurses. Ms. Breslin also contributed to the revision of *Guidelines for Construction and Equipment for Medical and Healthcare Facilities,* a publication of the American Institute of Architects.

Gerry Brueckner, RN, MBA, is the administrator/AVP of the Baylor Center for Restorative Care and the Pediatric Center for Restorative Care, both in Dallas. Previously, she was administrator of Baylor Home Care. Gerry has been active in many health care organizations including the board of directors for the AHA Section on Aging and Long-Term Care and the board of directors of the National Association of Long-Term Care Hospitals; she served as the AHA representative on the JCAHO professional and technical advisory committee for home care. She has been active in the Society of Ambulatory Care Professionals and has given frequent talks on case management and continuum of care.

Dorothy A. Calabrese, RN, MSN, CURN, is a clinical nurse specialist in the Department of Medical/Surgical Nursing at the Cleveland Clinic Foundation. Her primary focus is urology/oncology patients. Previously, she was head nurse of the urology/gynecology nursing unit, a 36-bed inpatient unit. She lectures frequently on topics related to urology and urology/oncology, and is an active member of the American Urologic Association, Allied, serving on the newly formed Clinical Practice Committee and Patient/Community Education Committee.

Kathryn Cantey Church, MS, CEAP, is employed by the United States Office of Personnel Management in Washington, DC, as manager of the employee assistance program. Previously, she was employed as an employee assistance counselor with Montgomery General Hospital, providing EAP services for nine federal agencies. She has worked in the area of employee assistance for the past 11 years, in both the United States and Japan, and her clinical expertise includes marital, family, individual, and group therapy. Ms. Church has developed and conducted training courses internationally on a variety of topics, including stress management, AIDS, preretirement, team building, personal financial management, and conflict resolution. She is a member of the National Academy of Counselors and Family Therapists, Inc., and the Employee Assistance Professionals Association, Inc.

Patricia DeHof, RNC, MS, is a perinatal nurse supervisor in the Women's Healthcare Services Division of Caremark, Inc., in Baltimore. She was instrumental in the development of the women's health home care program in the Baltimore and Washington, DC, areas. Ms. DeHof also is a certified OB-GYN and adult nurse practitioner with 10 years' obstetric experience in hospitals, clinics, private practice, and home care. She currently is a member of AWHONN and Sigma Theta Tau.

Mary Lynn Droughton, RN, MSN, is a head and neck oncology clinical nurse specialist at Cleveland Clinic Career Center. Previously, she was an instructor in nursing education at Cleveland Clinic Foundation. Before that, Ms. Droughton was a plastic and reconstructive surgery clinical nurse.

Carol Wilson Garvey, MD, MPH, is in the private practice of family medicine in Montgomery County, Maryland, where she has served as president of the county medical society and both secretary and treasurer of the state medical society. Prior to entering private practice in 1978, she worked in a variety of settings including a community health center, a city hospital, a university health service, and a health maintenance organization. As a medical officer with the federal government for five years, she wrote and lectured on quality assurance for community health centers, state maternal and child health programs, and the federal family planning program, of which she served as deputy director. She holds clinical teaching appointments at Georgetown University and the George Washington University School of Medicine, in Washington, DC.

Talar Glover, RN, MS, CNS is quality assurance/education coordinator at Baylor Center for Restorative Care, in Dallas. She is coeditor of *Decision Making in Gerontologic Nursing* (Mosby Year Book, 1993). Previously, she was director of medical/surgical nursing at Humana Hospital Medical City, also in Dallas.

Eileen Smyth Groh, RN, MSN, is an outpatient clinical coordinator in the Department of Hematology and Medical Oncology at the Cleveland Clinic Foundation. Previously, she was a clinical nurse specialist (palliative care service) and a urologic oncology nurse at the Cleveland Clinic Foundation.

Mary Ann House-Fancher, ARNP, MSN, CCRN, is a cardiovascular coordinator at Shands Hospital in Gainesville, Florida. Previously, she was an assistant professor in the University of Florida Graduate Nursing Program. She also was a cath lab director in the Division of Cardiology, Holmes Regional Medical Center, in Melbourne, Florida.

Samuel J. Kiehl III, MD, is director of emergency services of Riverside Methodist Hospitals, chief executive officer and president of Olentangy Emergency Physicians, and CEO of Physicians Professional Management Corporation, in Columbus, Ohio. He serves as an assistant clinical professor in the Department of Emergency Medicine and medical director of Pleasant Township Fire Department. Previously, he served on the board of directors of the Ohio Chapter of the American College of Emergency Physicians and was medical director of the Washington-Perry Fire Department.

Dawn Lajeunesse, BSN, MS, is a writer/consultant and owner of Professional Communication Services in Albany, New York. Her previous positions include director of human resources and quality assurance at the Visiting Nurse Service Association of Schenectady County, in New York, director of nursing at the VNA of Albany, and regional manager for Upjohn Healthcare Services. She has 23 years' experience in home health care.

Judith A. Lebanowski is founding executive director of Hospice at Riverside and past president of the Ohio Hospice Organization. She is affiliated with Riverside Methodist Hospitals in Columbus, Ohio, Hospice at Riverside, which operates a freestanding hospice care facility providing home care, day care, inpatient care, and bereavement services to terminally ill persons and their families. Ms. Lebanowski has been active in the development of hospice care in Ohio since 1980.

Gail P. Loadman, RN, CEN, is director of nursing, emergency services, at Riverside Methodist Hospitals, in Columbus, Ohio. Ms. Loadman is affiliated with the Emergency Nurse Association and ENCARE.

Linda Waite Maurano, BSN, MSN, is president and chief executive of the Visiting Nurse Association of Washington, DC, and senior vice-president of Medlantic Enterprises Inc., which manages a full scope of alternate site health care businesses. Previously, she was vice-president of Child Ventures, Inc., a subsidiary of Children's National Medical Center and executive director of Children's Home Health Care Services, in Washington, DC. While at Children's Ms. Maurano managed five pediatric licensed, certified, and JCAHO-accredited businesses servicing a tri-state area: a home health agency, a private duty agency, a hospice, home medical equipment, and home infusion. She also is adjunct faculty in the Graduate School of Nursing at The Catholic University of America and clinical instructor in the School of Nursing at Georgetown University. Additionally, she has served on the board of directors of Capital Home Health Association and Child Health Corporation of America. Ms. Maurano has served the home care industry for the past 22 years and actively publishes in the field of home health and management.

Arthur M. Melvin, MHA, NCADC, CEAP, is director for substance abuse treatment services at Providence Hospital, in Washington, DC. Additionally, he is responsible for delivery of counseling services and program planning for Seton House, the addiction recovery program at Providence Hospital. He has served on the executive boards of the District of Columbia Professional Alcoholism and Drug Abuse Counselors' Association and the District of Columbia Counselors Certification Board.

David P. Moxley, PhD, is associate professor of social work at Wayne State University, in Detroit. A former mental health administrator, Dr. Moxley is author of _The Practice of Case Management_ (Sage, 1989).

Marcie Parker, MA, MPA, CFLE, currently works full time in managed care for the aged for a major corporation and also is a doctoral student in family social science at the University of Minnesota. She is widely published in managed care, aging, long-term care, health care, and case management.

Previously, Ms. Parker served for six years as senior research associate with InterStudy's Center for Aging and Long-Term Care; as executive director of a statewide training and education program on all aspects of aging; as survey manager for a migrant council; and as director of admissions and discharge planning and research for an innovative skilled nursing facility. In addition, she has held a variety of academic and teaching positions and has given a number of workshops and presentations at state and national meetings.

Margaret E. Piazza, LCSW-C, BSN, MSW, is clinical social worker/patient education coordinator in the AIDS Service Diagnostic Evaluation Unit of the Division of Infectious Diseases at Johns Hopkins University School of Medicine, in Baltimore. Her experience in community health includes serving as coordinator of the U.S. Navy PEERS Program, which provides training and support for families at risk of abuse and neglect. She has four and a half years' experience in clinical social work service with HIV/AIDS patients. Ms. Piazza also has edited a quarterly newsletter as well as informational brochures.

Susan C. Rucker, MSW, MEd, is a clinical social worker and manager in the AIDS Service Diagnostic Evaluation Unit of the Division of Infectious Diseases at Johns Hopkins University School of Medicine, in Baltimore. She has five years' medical social work service at Johns Hopkins Hospital in surgery, psychiatry, and medicine. She also has five years' experience with the AIDS service providing direct clinical services to HIV patients.

Elaine M. Sampson, MS, RN, is vice-president of marketing and new business development at The Visiting Nurse Association of Chicago.

Steven Sieverts, MS, is an independent management consultant in managed health care, working in both the United States and the United Kingdom. In 1994, he retired early as a senior officer from Blue Cross and Blue Shield of the National Capital Area in Washington, DC, where he had served since 1985. Previously, he held a similar position with Empire Blue Cross and Blue Shield in New York. He has served as CEO of a major teaching hospital in Philadelphia and as head of the areawide health planning agency in Pittsburgh. Mr. Sieverts studied hospital administration at Columbia University in New York City and today holds the position of adjunct associate professor at Georgetown University School of Medicine in Washington, DC.

James A. Sliwa, DO, is associate professor, Department of Physical Medicine and Rehabilitation at Northwestern University Medical School, in Chicago, and an attending physician at the Rehabilitation Institute of Chicago (RIC). He is director of general rehabilitation and director of residency training at RIC.

Roger B. Upson, PhD, is Minnesota Care Officer and Physician Clinic Consultant, HealthSpan Corporation, in Minneapolis. Previously he was senior vice-president of the managed care division of Health One Corporation in Minneapolis. Dr. Upson served as chief financial officer of American Medcenters, Inc. (an HMO management company), and Park Nicollet Medical Center (a multispecialty group practice). He also was professor of finance and director of MBA programs at the University of Minnesota.

Cherie Weber, MS, RN, is division director for community health services at Illinois Valley Community Hospital in Peru, Illinois. Having worked in hospital home care since 1979, Ms. Weber currently is responsible for the administration of home health services, Medicare hospice services, private duty agency services, an adult day center, and numerous community health promotional activities. She delivers frequent national and local presentations in all areas of home care administration and staff retention. Previously, she was director of nursing and special projects coordinator for nurse recruitment and retention for the Illinois Hospital Association.

Foreword

Informative and comprehensive, *Outpatient Case Management: Strategies for a New Reality* enters the health care reform literature as a seminal work. The book defines, describes, and defends the use of case management as a highly transferable and effective approach for gluing together our current health care delivery system (or lack thereof!).

Outpatient Case Management includes information on specialty areas ranging from neonatology and pediatrics, emergency care, AIDS, and employee assistance programs, to hospices and long-term care. At all times, the authors are deeply grounded in the value of placing patients and families into a custom-designed, well-integrated set of multidisciplinary services. The reader will quickly learn how the generic case management process becomes a focused strategy for each type of outpatient experience.

The text mirrors the process it proposes by providing us with complete assessments of care systems, clarity of problem formulation and potential case management goals, specific design suggestions for achieving those goals, and insights into current and future issues. We not only receive a thorough consultation, such as how hospitals can better serve their communities, but also are exposed to new or reframed ideas about insurers, physicians, funding, implementation barriers, and health care policy. Hot issues such as why nurses generally make the best case managers, how much control payers should have in case management, and whether cost reductions should always be the first priority of a case management model are tackled.

Readers at any level of experience with case management will learn from and enjoy this work. Although case management is a logical, commonsense model, the way the contributing authors have successfully applied it to diverse settings offers lessons for everyone. Thanks to both the contributors and the editors for giving us years' worth of synthesis and wisdom.

Karen Zander
The Center for Case Management
April 1994

Preface

A new era of health care is upon us. The stimulus and pace of reform is driving public policymakers and health care organizations to escalate efforts at redesigning our nation's health delivery system. Extraordinary pressure from the government, employers, and insurers to control medical costs remains the primary impetus in forging new directions for managing health and medical care. In these changing times, organizational success and financial viability will depend in large part on the response of individual organizations with innovative, coordinated, and interdisciplinary methods of care and resource management across a full-care continuum. Integrated health care systems and alternative care delivery models are replacing traditional delivery arrangements, thus effecting a more organized, seamless continuum of diagnostic and therapeutic services.

In this milieu, outpatient case management will emerge as an essential and prominent feature of our restructured care delivery system. Overall, the rubric of case management embraces numerous models of interdisciplinary care management. Although often emulated or described under separate banners such as care mapping, recovery paths, critical pathways, or target tracks, these focused, collaborative applications present intrinsic and strategic value to outcome-based care management. More than sophisticated theory, the practice of case management offers established merit as a master link in coordinating variable chains of services and programs. Further, and more important, case management's focus on bringing patients and their families to appropriate levels of the care continuum offers a preeminent strategy for patient/family advocacy, quality of care, and cost savings.

Although the concept and practice of case management is not new, there is growing appreciation of its position and value in the contemporary outpatient arena. As the current shift from inpatient to outpatient care accelerates, new challenges are arising for consumers, health care providers, practitioners, and organizational leaders alike. In the ambulatory environment, for example, our aging and elderly population often requires access to multiple services, systems, and providers in order to receive prescribed levels of diagnostic, therapeutic, or definitive care. This growing and conspicuous demand for services has precipitated an increasingly complex and fragmented health care landscape. In today's dynamic marketplace, outpatient case management is a fundamental component in the reengineering of health delivery systems.

This publication defines the numerous and intricate parameters of outpatient case management and illustrates its benefits within a framework of health care reform. Part one addresses the benefits and salient features of case management, establishes a premise for an integrated system approach to achieving a seamless continuum of care, discusses various components of program development, and ultimately categorizes the various programmatic prototypes. Chapter 1 presents an overview of a dynamic health care industry in the throes of transition. In a unique characterization of the outpatient care arena that explains evolving trends and industry direction, the chapter espouses a reality-based approach to a newly restructured health delivery system. Inherent in this forecast is the very real and significant need for case management programs as an innovative response to outpatient care management. Chapter 2 offers global insight into the definition, concept, and practice of case management in contemporary times. It provides an in-depth look at the need for, and benefits of, integrated outpatient case management programs in an increasingly complex care continuum. Chapter 3 discusses in detail the special considerations and components of outpatient case management from the payer's perspective. Chapter 4 looks at the planning agenda, needs assessment, and other special considerations for developing case management programs. Chapter 5 introduces various professional behaviors and strategies that must be addressed in order to achieve successful program development and outcomes. Chapters 6 and 7 discuss the role, function, and process of case management in linking clients with systems to achieve optimum outcomes and access to the continuum of care. Part one emphasizes the function of customary practice models and the case manager as the primary care coordinator.

Part two presents 16 case models of outpatient case management programs. Each chapter describes how a specific outpatient case management model works and provides an example of a successful program. Further, each program illustration depicts a specific consumer population and offers insight into special needs generated by virtue of patient age, level of handicap, or skilled care and technology requirements. Many of the models discuss barriers to implementation as well as the intricacies of coordinating and ensuring care delivery in the outpatient setting. An annotated bibliography is appended to acquaint the reader with selective texts and journal literature related to case management and issues surrounding program implementation. Given the merits, intricacies, and diversity of case management programs, the bibliography offers readers a valuable resource for additional information and guidance. In its culmination, this publication suggests an infrastructure for health reform with a humanized approach to an administration-driven system. It champions a framework for health care delivery that reduces service fragmentation and slows cost escalation, while addressing the primary service needs of consumers with a process of dedicated advocacy.

Michelle Regan Donovan
Theodore A. Matson
March 1994

Acknowledgments

The editors, Ted Matson and Michelle Regan Donovan, wish to thank and acknowledge the many individuals whose contributions and dedicated efforts made this book a reality. We extend special appreciation to the individual chapter authors, whose knowledge, practical experience, and willingness to share are the essence of this publication. Special thanks also to the editorial staff of American Hospital Publishing, Inc.; especially Audrey Kaufman, project editor, for her invaluable commentary, editorial assistance, and enthusiastic project oversight. Thanks also go to Marlene Chamberlain, formerly of AHPI, for her encouragement during project conception and initiation.

Ted and Michelle wish to offer special recognition and thanks to Karen Zander for her pioneering efforts in case management in the acute care setting. Her dedication to and integration of the process of patient care has offered significant structure to the future of health care.

In addition, Michelle Donovan would like to offer special appreciation and recognition to coeditor Ted Matson for his vision, foresight, and undying affinity for ambulatory care; to Mary Gavin, Paul Smith, and Shirley Inniss, who offered a lifetime of invaluable learning experiences; to John Kernan III for mind preservation with computer and moral support; to Lisa, Tom, and Jennifer Donovan for understanding what "quiet time" means; and to Chuck Miller for offering balance, frivolity, and editorial and computer expertise. Finally, Michelle would like to thank her parents, Faye and Jim Regan, for their investment of lifelong love, encouragement, and pride.

Part I

Chapter 1

The Changing Environment of Outpatient Care

Theodore A. Matson

• Introduction

Without question, the health care industry is in the early stages of a massive transformation that will forever alter many traditional patterns of patient care delivery. It is expected that case management will play a pivotal role in this new environment. Although outpatient care — the delivery of services to patients who do not occupy inpatient beds and do not require 24-hour care — has always been an important facet of the health care continuum, it undoubtedly will become a leading force in future restructuring efforts. For many providers, inpatient care has matured or stabilized — a trend that for all intents and purposes will never be reversed.

Although case management has been defined, prescribed, debated, and utilized for a seemingly inexhaustible array of patient services, its true meaning and effective application are still widely misunderstood. For each professional or provider type, the words *case management* seem to denote a different purpose, scope, and function of service provision.

As the health care industry continues to cut costs, increase operational efficiency, and pursue different forms of integrated delivery arrangements, case management in the outpatient sector will be valued for three primary purposes: (1) to improve the patient care process associated with traditional forms of outpatient services; (2) to support the movement to substitute outpatient encounters for inpatient stays; and (3) to integrate traditional as well as new outpatient regimens with nonhospital providers to effect seamless continuums of diagnostic and therapeutic service delivery. This flurry of activity in the outpatient arena will have profound implications for all institutions and providers, which for decades have evolved around a system devoted primarily to acute care.

This chapter describes some of the cost reduction initiatives currently in place that are changing the dynamics of the health care marketplace. It also discusses the role of outpatient care and the value of outpatient case management within this new environment.

• Changing Marketplace Dynamics

Today, hospitals derive approximately 30 percent of their net revenues from outpatient services. Although numerous institutions have witnessed double-digit growth in outpatient care during the past several years and some expect outpatients to contribute 50 percent of net revenues by the end of this decade, many have not seriously committed their organizations to prepare for this reality; in fact, fewer than 20 percent of our nation's health care institutions have established a position of authority to oversee their ambulatory services.[1]

For years, the literature has trumpeted the coming of cost controls, consolidation, integration, and managed care initiatives to tame a system out of control and fraught with abuse. Although many have recognized the merits of controlling system expenditures, few could have imagined the rapidity with which such changes are currently taking place and, further, the degree to which some providers are altering the health care landscape.

To appreciate the effect of these rapid and profound changes, as well as the ultimate challenges these developments will pose in a new health care system that embraces outpatient care, a number of industry developments are noteworthy of review. Following are examples of efforts that employers, providers, and payers are currently pursuing, either independently or collaboratively, to reduce the cost of care.

- After experiencing health care cost increases of 8 to 12 percent in 1992, nearly a dozen of the largest employers in the U.S. reported a significant slowdown in growth rates in 1993. As a result of greater utilization of managed care programs, direct contracting with efficient providers of services, centralized review systems that limit the use of costly medical services, and programs that reimburse for outpatient versus inpatient care, a number of employers now are experiencing increases of 6 to 9 percent.[2]
- Despite the success of some companies in slowing their health care cost increases, many others continue to experience rapid rates of growth. This has resulted in greater out-of-pocket expenses for thousands of employees and in company layoffs, particularly when charges must be taken against corporate earnings to pay for funding of retiree health care benefits. To help defray its double-digit cost increases, DuPont has increased its employees' out-of-pocket contributions from 11 to 20 percent; by 1997, any health care cost increases will be split fifty-fifty by the company and plan members, both active and retired.[3]
- Nearly 140 million employees in the U.S. are covered by corporate health plans, yet until recently they have had little incentive or knowledge to judge the pricing of alternative coverage plans. With higher deductibles and copayments associated with care rendered, many patients are beginning to comparison shop for services. For example, employees at NCR Corporation have

access to the company's fee schedule, which shows what the company plan will pay for more than 11,000 procedures, giving patients the opportunity to discuss fees with physicians prior to receiving any procedure or service.[4]

- Clinical practice guidelines to curtail overutilization of services during the course of a patient's diagnosis and treatment are increasingly being mandated. Blue Cross and Blue Shield of Illinois now requires physician specialists to follow clinical guidelines for 14 procedures. The state of Maine has instituted physician guidelines that, if followed, will also provide malpractice relief.[5,6]

- Although home infusion therapy costs less than similar services provided in the inpatient setting, insurers are targeting providers of these services to effect even lower rates of reimbursement. Thus, with their impressive buying clout, health insurance concerns are able to effect direct contracting arrangements with a limited number of providers to significantly reduce financial outlays. Through such arrangements, Massachusetts Blue Cross estimates that home infusion therapy expenses for its 2.4 million members will decrease from $20 to $10 million—a savings of 50 percent annually.[7]

- Medicare continues to develop bundled payment demonstration projects to ultimately slow the cost of financial outlays for high-volume services. In the much-touted cardiac bypass surgery demonstration project, Medicare negotiated 8 to 20 percent discounts in payments to providers. Recently, a similar system was initiated for cataract surgery—the most common surgical procedure performed, primarily on an outpatient basis, on Americans over 65 years old. In 1991, Medicare paid $3.4 billion for 1.35 million cataract surgeries.[8]

- For-profit entities, which claim to provide outpatient services at costs that are 30 to 40 percent lower than those of their hospital counterparts, are experiencing an erosion of patient referrals and revenues due to negotiated arrangements of prepaid health care plans. For example, Medical Imaging Centers of America, which operates nearly 250 diagnostic imaging centers/mobile units, reported a net loss of $20.3 million in 1992 versus a net loss of $10.4 million in 1991—an increase of nearly 100 percent in one year.[9] Similarly, Maxum Health Corporation, which operates nearly 70 imaging units/centers in 23 states, reported a net loss of $8.3 million in 1992 compared to a net loss of $1 million in 1991—an increase of more than 700 percent in one year.[10]

- Following management practices learned in other industries, many institutions and providers have begun to apply total quality management principles and patient pathways to increase the efficiency of the patient care process. Although recent developments, many of these innovative practices are significantly reducing lengths of stay (LOS), and thus costs of care, for specific diagnoses and patient types. Henry Ford Health System, in Detroit, developed protocols to shorten LOS to one day for 80

percent of certain cancer patients requiring chemotherapy—patients who previously were hospitalized for three to four days.[11]
- According to a survey by the actuarial firm of Milliman & Robertson, 24 percent of hospital admissions and 29 percent of inpatient days are medically unnecessary. If operational inefficiencies and other factors were eliminated, the researchers concluded, hospitals could achieve an average of 200 to 255 inpatient days per 1,000 population versus today's national average of 480 inpatient days per 1,000 population.[12]
- Many companies are developing their own primary care and specialty clinics to directly provide health care for employees, a concept unheard of only a few years ago. In November 1993, Aetna Life Insurance Company established five primary care centers in Atlanta, with plans to develop others in the metropolitan markets of Charlotte, North Carolina; Chicago; Dallas–Fort Worth; and Washington–Baltimore. Open to all residents of each community, the centers have a threefold mission: (1) to contain rising health care costs, (2) to improve patient access to primary care in underserved areas, and (3) to manage the overall patient care process and improve quality of services.[13]
- Some companies have opted to develop health care satellites in collaboration with major care providers. In January 1993, the Mayo Clinic and John Deere, the large farm equipment manufacturer, collaborated on development of a primary care satellite to provide care for approximately 35,000 John Deere employees in Moline, Illinois. Citing the goal to develop "a continuous system of care from family practice to the specialty level," Mayo physicians will directly provide specialty services that are not locally available to plan enrollees who receive care at the clinic. Mayo also has initiated a similar clinic system for 30,000 John Deere employees in Waterloo, Iowa.[14]
- The ever-rising number of mergers and acquisitions among health care institutions and provider groups portends massive infrastructure changes for U.S. hospitals and the communities they serve. In a recent study of hospital mergers, the American Hospital Association's Research and Educational Trust revealed that 52 percent of the hospitals involved in mergers between 1983 and 1988 dropped acute care services.[15]
- In the physician provider community, reform efforts and the need for system integration have spawned more mergers, affiliations, and acquisitions. In September 1992, Hawthorne Medical Group, in Los Angeles, and Mullikin Medical Center, in Artesia, California, announced plans to merge, creating one of the top 20 medical groups in the U.S. On a lesser scale but equally important, in early 1993 Sharp Healthcare, in San Diego, affiliated with Mission Park Medical Clinic, a physician group practice composed of 88 professionals providing services at five family practice, pediatric, and urgent care clinics in the San Diego metropolitan area.[16,17]
- The realm of such infrastructure change is wide-ranging. The Cleveland Clinic, in Cleveland, has agreed to allow the physicians of Kaiser Permanente

of Ohio to provide care for its enrolled population of 200,000 at the clinic's acute care facility. And in the Boston metropolitan area, the Lahey Clinic, composed of nearly 300 physicians, has embarked on a strategy of mergers, acquisitions, and affiliations with suburban hospitals and other group practices. In October 1992, Lahey announced plans to acquire a 59-bed acute care facility in the North Shore area of Boston and to convert it into a five-story, 140,000-square-foot ambulatory services complex.[18,19]

• The '90s: The Decade to Confront Outpatient Care

Clearly, the movement to reform the health care system has already begun with much fervor and force. Despite the ultimate outcome of major policy initiatives and their level of actual implementation, marketplace dynamics will continue to effect industry change. As costs are reined in, alliances of providers developed, and the efficiencies of systemwide operations realized, health care organizations will aggressively pursue the most appropriate forms of service delivery. It is within this context that the role of outpatient care — and the value of outpatient case management — must be discussed.

Positioning for Change

Although it has been promised for years, the real shift to outpatient care has not yet been fully realized. However, by the end of this decade, it is conceivable that 30 to 40 percent of traditional admissions will shift to outpatient encounters. The reasons for this shift are actually quite simple:

1. Changing patient demographics
2. Stricter payer initiatives
3. Technological advances

Technology will have perhaps the greatest impact on patient care because noninvasive and minimally invasive procedures and services will be favored for their role in reducing the cost and perhaps necessity of an inpatient admission. Concomitantly, as payers continue to adopt outpatient alternatives, financial performance will be greatly affected. Thus, outpatient care will increasingly drive overall profitability and may ultimately determine an institution's success or failure.[20]

To succeed in the approaching structural reorganization of outpatient care, a long-term strategy will be required. Building on the diversification activities of the past two decades, today's marketplace must reposition its resources and realign its delivery systems to effectively meet outpatient care needs. Such reality-based planning will require the in-depth analysis, development, and enhancement of four strategic components. These include:[21]

1. Creating a dynamic organizational structure(s) that favors an outpatient versus inpatient care orientation
2. Emphasizing hospital-based outpatient arrangements, including priority attention to functional, system, and physical redesign efforts
3. Achieving excellence in developing an infrastructure of primary care providers
4. Implementing demand-specific specialty outreach services, whether developed in hospital-affiliated, freestanding, and/or home ambulatory settings

Understanding the New Technological Reality

The move away from inpatient and toward outpatient care will have enormous implications and repercussions. Technology and its application will be largely responsible for this continuing shift, and the new environment will merely reflect what we have been experiencing for some time—a growing understanding of the true role and dimensions of technology.

The very definition of *technology* has changed in the past two decades. It used to mean equipment-related advances; however, technology now includes not only amazingly sophisticated equipment but also new techniques, medical and surgical procedures, therapies, and all sorts of drugs and devices. In the future, these advances and developments will have a particularly strong impact on cardiovascular and cancer services. Most institutions will no doubt perform the majority of diagnostic cardiac catheterizations on an outpatient basis. Additionally, nearly 90 percent of cancer-related services will be performed in the outpatient setting.[22]

From a programmatic perspective, the single largest trend for outpatient care in the future will be the movement to minimally invasive care and surgical care. Since the introduction of fiber-optic scopes in the 1970s, researchers, developers, and manufacturers have made technologic leaps and bounds in the direct visualization of internal body cavities. For instance, fiber-optic approaches for visualization of the digestive tract have significantly improved the diagnosis and treatment of digestive disorders. A number of endoscopic programs have since expanded their offerings to include therapeutic approaches such as locating and removing polyps. Other fiber-optic uses have expanded to revolutionize the field of orthopedic care. Fiber-optic technology is now being used in all phases of orthopedics and has become the diagnostic tool of choice for shoulder and knee injuries. Further, over the past several years, operative laparascopes for use in cholecystectomies, appendectomies, nephrectomies, and hysterectomies have brought about a fundamental shift in the way general surgery is performed. Overall, these and other advances in technologies make it clear that minimally invasive approaches to patient diagnosis and management will quickly become the preferred standard.[23]

Adjusting to the Operational Challenges of Systemwide Restructuring

Although day-to-day operational considerations will occupy their outpatient management concerns, providers also will be faced with a dilemma: Should services be expanded within the confines of an existing hospital facility, or should certain services be unbundled into freestanding campus or remote facilities? The decision will be difficult.

Because numerous players are involved and turf issues are often greatest in the outpatient arena, each institution will have to find its own appropriate course of action. But outpatient service delivery will surely figure prominently in every provider's agenda for the next several years. To understand the implications of pursuing future outpatient initiatives and the promise of achieving operational efficiency to lower the costs of care, it is appropriate to quantify the most likely responses to marketplace restructuring efforts as follows:

- As outpatient programs and services proliferate, most hospitals will have no other choice than to physically separate outpatients from inpatient settings. A major focus on facilities devoted exclusively to the unique needs of outpatients will be necessary; medical–surgical procedural and short-stay services will be the area of greatest expansion.
- As hospitals make large-scale commitments to outpatient settings, physicians and physician groups will increasingly seek to practice in these settings for a number of reasons, including the need for an increased market share of patients, enhanced payer mix of patients, opportunities for managed care, convenience to hospital services and technologies, and practice management support.
- As marketplace dynamics accelerate, development of freestanding facilities will be curtailed. Overcapacity in some markets will lead to selective consolidation because multispecialty arrangements will intensify. Further, comprehensive freestanding ambulatory care developments will require a multidimensional array of services to achieve utilization and financial viability. Although specific types of facilities such as primary care clinics and occupational health centers will continue to be developed, many other prototypes will only be applicable to specialized markets.

Redefining Outpatient Care

The many services provided along the outpatient care continuum reflect the diversity of today's fragmented and complex delivery arrangements. Coordinating these multifaceted offerings will require management flexibility and commitment to the overall case management process. As the variety of our program models indicate, the case management function is highly individualized and not necessarily applicable across the continuum of services.

From the outset, the evolving role of outpatient case management will include care delivery in four distinct settings. These are:

1. Physician office settings, regardless of organizational sponsorship or ownership
2. Hospital-based departments and campus facilities
3. Myriad other freestanding outpatient settings, including the full range of diagnostic and therapeutic centers
4. Services provided by home care professionals and related providers

In view of the hospital's continued orientation as the hub of the outpatient care continuum, it is likely that case management efforts will be centralized, at least conceptually. To this end, hospitals have clearly begun to respond with innovative approaches for increasing the efficiency of the patient care process. Again, the wide variety of case management applications for specific outpatient programs, as illustrated in our program models, attests to the degree to which such innovations already have been implemented.

Although individualized approaches are indeed important, providers must anticipate that, again, because the large-scale movement to outpatient care is not yet complete, management directives in case management will continue to change. In other words, today's coordinated care management programs have been designed primarily for today's outpatients and will have to be refined for the many patients who will soon be shifted from inpatient stays to outpatient encounters.

To illustrate this point, a sample listing of various inpatient diagnoses with average lengths of stay (ALOS) of one to two days is provided in figure 1-1. Although the mix of patient types will be different for each institution, it is widely acknowledged that short-stay care admissions will soon fall under the purview of the outpatient setting. Typically, these short-stay admissions represent at least 25 percent of a hospital's total patient days; for some, they may represent up to 40 percent of total patient days.[24]

In essence, the movement to short-stay services will redefine outpatient care in hospitals, both conceptually and programmatically. This reality already is apparent to the many institutions that have developed early admission units and alternate care units to expedite the initial processing, disposition, and early discharge of specific patient types—for example, those undergoing diagnostic cardiac catheterization and those requiring short-term recovery from surgical procedures such as laparoscopic cholecystectomy.

Figure 1-1. Short-Stay Inpatient Admissions, by Diagnosis, That May Soon Shift to the Outpatient Arena

Code	Diagnosis	Code	Diagnosis
075	INFECTIOUS MONONUCLEOSIS	9685	POIS-TOPIC/INFILT ANESTH
2353	UNC BEHAV NEO LIVER	9712	POISON-SYMPATHOMIMETICS
23770	NEUROFIBROMATOSIS, UNSPE	9726	POIS-ANTIHYPERTEN AGENT
2535	DIABETES INSIPIDUS	9757	POISONING-ANTIASTHMATICS
2707	STRAIG AMIN-ACID MET NEC	981	TOXIC EFF PETROLEUM PROD
3229	MENINGITIS NOS	9876	TOXIC EFF CHLORINE GAS
33181	REYE'S SYNDROME	9890	TOXIC EFFECT CYANIDES
4640	ACUTE LARYNGITIS	9893	TOX EFF ORGANPHOS/CARBAM
49301	EXT ASTHMA W STATUS ASTH	9940	EFFECTS OF LIGHTNING
5692	RECTAL ANAL STENOSIS	38650	LABRYINTHINE DYSFUNC NOS
7804	DIZZINESS AND GIDDINESS	41041	INFERIOR MI INITIAL CARE
7861	STRIDOR	4413	RUPT ABD AORTIC ANEURYSM
8500	CONCUSSION W/O COMA	4439	PERIPH VASCULAR DIS NOS
8501	CONCUSSION-BRIEF COMA	53500	ACT GAST W/O HEMORRHAGE
8509	CONCUSSION NOS	5920	CALCULUS OF KIDNEY
85402	BRAIN INJ NEC-BRIEF COMA	7244	LUMBOSACRAL NEURITIS NOS
9070	LT EFF INTRACRANIAL INJ	72709	SYNOVITIS NEC
9695	POISON-TRANQUILIZER NEC	7840	HEADACHE
9713	POISONING-SYMPATHOLYTICS	87349	OPEN WOUND OF FACE NEC
9870	TOXIC EFF LIQ PETROL GAS	94129	2ND DEG BURN HEAD-MULT
9893	TOX EFF ORGANPHOS/CARBAM	9680	POIS-CNS MUSCLE DEPRESS
9941	DROWNING/NONFATAL SUBMER	9690	POISONING-ANTIDEPRESSANT
0093	DIARRHEA OF INFECT ORIG	9694	POIS-BENZODIAZEPINE TRAN
07051	HEP C W/O HEP COMA	9757	POISONING-ANTIASTHMATICS
22800	HEMANGIOMA NOS	9874	TOXIC EFFECT FREON
2874	SECOND THROMBOCYTOPENIA	44022	ATHEROSCL EXTREM W/REST
2893	LYMPHADENITIS NOS	26	RADIOLOGY
30500	ALCOHOL ABUSE-UNSPEC	4377	TRANSIENT GLOBAL AMNESIA
30502	ALCOHOL ABUSE-EPISODIC	7870	NAUSEA AND VOMITING
311	DEPRESSIVE DISORDER NEC	1419	MALIG NEO TONGUE NOS
3336	IDIOPAT TORSION DYSTONIA	1941	MALIG NEO PARATHYROID
4441	THORACIC AORTIC EMBOLISM	20008	RETICULOSARCOMA MULT
44421	UPPER EXTREMITY EMBOLISM	2148	LIPOMA NEC
45981	VENOUS INSUFFICIENCY NOS	2300	CA IN SITU ORAL CAV/PHAR
5643	VOMITING POST-GI SURGERY	2397	ENDOCRINE/NERV NEO NOS
5649	FUNCT DIS INTESTINE NOS	2891	CHRONIC LYMPHADENITIS
5650	ANAL FISSURE	3102	POSTCONCUSSION SYNDROME
56949	RECTAL ANAL DIS NEC	36960	BLINDNESS. ONE EYE
V725	RADIOLOGICAL EXAM NEC	40290	HYPERTENSIVE HRT DIS NOS
78551	CARDIOGENIC SHOCK	4440	ABD AORTIC EMBOLISM
86101	HEART CONTUSION-CLOSED	4519	THROMBOPHLEBITIS NOS
9221	CONTUSION OF CHEST WALL	4550	INT HEMORRHOID W/O COMPL
9630	POIS-ANTIALLRG/ANTIEMET	4558	HEMRRHOID NOS W COMP NEC
96500	POISONING-OPIUM NOS	45989	CIRCULATORY DISEASE NEC
9651	POISONING-SALICYLATES	462	ACUTE PHARYNGITIS
9663	POIS-ANTICONVUL NEC/NOS	5190	TRACHEOSTOMY COMPLIC

(Continued on next page)

Figure 1-1. (Continued)

Code	Diagnosis	Code	Diagnosis
5529	HERNIA. SITE NOS W OBSTR	80220	MANDIBLE FX NOS-CLOSED
56039	IMPACTION INTESTINE NEC	80301	CL SKULL FX NEC W/O COMA
56949	RECTAL ANAL DIS NEC	80340	CL SKL FX NEC/BR INJ NEC
5759	DIS OF GALLBLADDER NOS	83905	DISLOC 5TH CERV VERT-CL
5921	CALCULUS OF URETER	8509	CONCUSSION NOS
5991	URETHRAL FISTULA	85409	BRAIN INJ NEC-CONCUSSION
61172	LUMP OR MASS IN BREAST	87342	OPEN WOUND OF FOREHEAD
6145	AC PELV PERITONITIS-FEM	95200	C1-C4 SPIN CORD INJ NOS
6146	FEM PELVIC PERITON ADHES	99672	OTH COMP CARDIAC DEVICE
6164	ABSCESS OF VULVA NEC	3320	PARALYSIS AGITANS
7092	SCAR FIBROSIS OF SKIN	5070	FOOD/VOMIT PNEUMONITIS
72743	GANGLION NOS	V548	ORTHOPEDIC AFTERCARE NEC
7803	CONVULSIONS	V725	RADIOLOGICAL EXAM NEC
78650	CHEST PAIN NOS	71618	TRAUM ARTHROPATHY NEC
7866	CHEST SWELLING/MASS/LUMP	7179	INT DERANGEMENT KNEE NOS
81601	FX MID/PRX PHAL. HAND-CL	71887	JT DERANGEMENT NEC-ANKLE
8470	SPRAIN OF NECK	71941	JOINT PAIN-SHLDER
8509	CONCUSSION NOS	71943	JOINT PAIN-FOREARM
85401	BRAIN INJURY NEC-NO COMA	72610	ROTATOR CUFF SYND NOS
86389	GI INJURY NEC-CLOSED	72767	RUPTURE ACHILLES TENDON
88000	OPEN WOUND OF SHOULDER	7295	PAIN IN LIMB
8840	OPEN WOUND ARM MULT/NOS	7352	HALLUX RIGIDUS
9118	SUPERFIC INJ TRUNK NEC	73679	ACQ ANKLE-FOOT DEF NEC
9190	ABRASION NEC	81213	FX GR TUBEROS HUMER-OPEN
9972	SURG COMP-PERI VASC SYST	81220	FX HUMERUS NOS-CLOSED
4149	CHR ISCHEMIC HRT DIS NOS	81221	FX HUMERUS SHAFT-CLOSED
4411	RUPTUR THORACIC ANEURYSM	81243	FX HUMER. MED CONDYL-CL
V533	ADJUST CARDIAC PACEMAKER	81303	MONTEGGIA'S FX-CLOSED
V725	RADIOLOGICAL EXAM NEC	81307	FX UP RADIUS NEC/NOS-CL
7847	EPISTAXIS	81342	FX DISTAL RADIUS NEC-CL
36510	OPEN-ANGLE GLAUCOMA NOS	81344	FX LOW RADIUS W ULNA-CL
3669	CATARACT NOS	81353	FX DISTAL ULNA-OPEN
42731	ATRIAL FIBRILLATION	81400	FX CARPAL BONE NOS-CLOSE
2120	BEN NEO NASAL CAV/SINUS	81502	FX METACARP BASE NEC-CL
2409	GOITER NOS	81509	MULT FX METACARPUS-CLOSE
2410	NONTOX UNINODULAR GOITER	8171	MULTIPLE FX HAND-OPEN
4611	AC FRONTAL SINUSITIS	83104	DISLOC ACROMIOCLAVIC-CL
470	DEVIATED NASAL SEPTUM	8399	DISLOCATION NEC-OPEN
4731	CHR FRONTAL SINUSITIS	8418	SPRAIN ELBOW/FOREARM NEC
4732	CHR ETHMOIDAL SINUSITIS	84200	SPRAIN OF WRIST NOS
4740	CHRONIC TONSILLITIS	87349	OPEN WOUND OF FACE NEC
47410	HYPERTROPHY T AND A	88102	OPEN WOUND OF WRIST
9330	FOREIGN BODY IN PHARYNX	9223	CONTUSION OF BACK
9933	CAISSON DISEASE	9594	HAND INJURY NOS
9951	ANGIONEUROTIC EDEMA	9974	SURG COMPLIC-GI TRACT
1917	MAL NEO BRAIN STEM	9988	SURGICAL COMPLICAT NEC
3529	CRANIAL NERVE DIS NOS	2102	BEN NEO MAJOR SALIVARY
73390	BONE CARTILAGE DIS NOS	4780	HYPERTRPH NASAL TURBINAT

Figure 1-1.   (Continued)

Code	Diagnosis	Code	Diagnosis
4781	NASAL SINUS DIS NEC	7803	CONVULSIONS
V524	FITTING BREAST PROSTHES	7890	ABDOMINAL PAIN
7090	DYSCHROMIA	85401	BRAIN INJURY NEC-NO COMA
74910	CLEFT LIP NOS	6179	ENDOMETRIOSIS NOS
7540	CONG SKULL/FACE/JAW DEF	64253	SEV PREECLAMP-ANTEPARTUM
78609	RESPIRATORY ABNORM NEC	65461	ABN CERVIX NEC-DELIVERED
85406	BRAIN INJ NEC-COMA NOS	66231	DELAY DEL 2ND TWIN-DELIV
87341	OPEN WOUND OF CHEEK	V240	POSTPART CARE AFTER DEL
8820	OPEN WOUND OF HAND	66404	DEL W 1 DEG LAC-POSTPART
2163	BENIGN NEO SKIN FACE NEC	66414	DEL W 2 DEG LAC-POSTPART
5252	ATROPHY ALVEOLAR RIDGE	V3101	TWIN LIVE,HOSP,W/ C-SECT
52689	JAW DISEASE NEC	0340	STREP SORE THROAT
8024	FX MALAR/MAXILLARY-CLOSE	2873	PRIMARY THROMBOCYTOPENIA
2337	CA IN SITU BLADDER	34510	GEN CONVUL EPIL W/O INTR
55090	UNILAT INGUINAL HERNIA	3469	MIGRAINE NOS
5640	CONSTIPATION	37610	CHR INFLAM NOS. ORBIT
59654	NEUROGENIC BLADDER, NOS	38010	INFEC OTITIS EXTERNA NOS
5991	URETHRAL FISTULA	4644	CROUP
5998	URINARY TRACT DIS NEC	4660	ACUTE BRONCHITIS
59984	OTHER SPEC URETHRA DISOR	4740	CHRONIC TONSILLITIS
60490	ORCHITIS/EPIDIDYMIT NOS	47410	HYPERTROPHY T AND A
60782	VASCULAR DISORDER. PENIS	515	POSTINFLAM PULM FIBROSIS
6081	SPERMATOCELE	51889	OTHER LUNG DISEASE NEC
7525	UNDESCENDED TESTICLE	53390	PEPTIC ULCER NOS
7526	MALE HYPOSPADIAS/EPISPAD	5362	PERSISTENT VOMITING
8782	OPN WOUND SCROTUM/TESTES	5370	ACQ PYLORIC STENOSIS
99639	MALFUNC GU DEV/GRAFT NEC	56039	IMPACTION INTESTINE NEC
4659	ACUTE URI NOS	5640	CONSTIPATION
61610	VAGINITIS NOS	5641	IRRITABLE COLON
6270	PREMENOPAUSE MENORRHAGIA	57420	CHOLELITHIASIS NOS
63711	ABORT NOS W HEMORR-INC	5798	INTEST MALABSORPTION NEC
8784	OPEN WOUND OF VULVA	5819	NEPHROTIC SYNDROME NOS
9973	SURG COMPLIC-RESPIR SYST	5881	NEPHROGEN DIABETES INSIP
63422	SPON AB W PEL DAMAG-COMP	V301	SINGL LIVEBRN-BEFORE ADM
63471	SPON AB W COMPL NEC-INC	7488	RESPIRATORY ANOMALY NEC
63570	LEG AB W COMPL NEC-UNSP	769	RESPIRATORY DISTRESS SYN
63572	LEG AB W COMPL NEC-COMP	7755	NEONATAL DEHYDRATION
63620	ILLEG AB W PEL DAMG-UNSP	7802	SYNCOPE AND COLLAPSE
63792	AB NOS UNCOMPLICAT-COMP	7821	NONSPECIF SKIN ERUPT NEC
65453	CERV INCOMPET-ANTEPARTUM	7842	SWELLING IN HEAD
2189	UTERINE LEIOMYOMA NOS	78600	RESPIRATORY ABNORM NOS
4661	ACUTE BRONCHIOLITIS	7862	COUGH
64000	THREATENED ABORT-UNSPEC	7891	HEPATOMEGALY
64003	THREATEN ABORT-ANTEPART	85400	BRAIN INJURY NEC
64183	ANTEPART HEM NEC-ANTEPAR	9661	POISON-HYDANTOIN DERIVAT
64193	ANTEPART HEM NOS-ANTEPAR	1574	MAL NEO ISLET LANGERHANS
64203	ESSEN HYPERTEN-ANTEPART	1624	MAL NEO MIDDLE LOBE LUNG1
66103	PRIM UTER INERT-ANTEPART	1978	SEC MAL NEO GI NEC

(Continued on next page)

Figure 1-1. (Continued)

Code	Diagnosis	Code	Diagnosis
2395	OTHER GU NEOPLASM NOS	78652	PAINFUL RESPIRATION
3094	ADJ REACT-EMOTION/CONDUC	30000	ANXIETY STATE NOS
3419	CNS DEMYELINATION NOS	34500	GEN NONCONVUL EPILEPSY
3462	VARIANTS OF MIGRAINE	37854	SIXTH NERVE PALSY
3510	BELL'S PALSY	4350	BASILAR ARTERY SYNDROME
36816	PSYCHOPHYSIC VISUAL DIST	72210	LUMBAR DISC DISPLACEMENT
38650	LABYRINTHINE DYSFUNC NOS	7289	MUSCLE/LIGAMENT DIS NOS
3963	MITRAL/AORTIC VAL INSUFF	7295	PAIN IN LIMB
41189	OTH ISCHEMIC HRT DIS	7814	TRANSIENT LIMB PARALYSIS
4251	HYPERTR OBSTR CARDIOMYOP	0049	SHIGELLOSIS NOS
4272	PAROX TACHYCARDIA NOS	0088	VIRAL ENTERITIS NOS
4292	ASCVD	0799	UNSP VIRAL/CHLAMYDIA INF
4371	AC CEREBROVASC INSUF NOS	1420	MALIG NEO PAROTID
4510	SUPERFIC PHLEBITIS-LEG	1431	MALIG NEO LOWER GUM
4552	INT HEMRRHOID W COMP NEC	1590	MALIG NEO INTESTINE NOS
4739	CHRONIC SINUSITIS NOS	1726	MALIG MELANOMA ARM
47870	DISEASE OF LARYNX NOS	1955	MALIGN NEOPL LEG
5206	TOOTH ERUPTION DISTURB	2141	LIPOMA SKIN NEC
55010	UNILAT ING HERNIA W OBST	2150	BEN NEO SOFT TISSUE HEAD
57450	CHOLEDOCHOLITHIASIS NOS	2271	BENIGN NEO PARATHYROID
5779	PANCREATIC DISEASE NOS	2298	BENIGN NEOPLASM NEC
V078	PROPHYLACTIC MEASURE NEC	2410	NONTOX UNINODULAR GOITER
V728	EXAMINATION NEC	2419	NONTOX NODUL GOITER NOS
7088	URTICARIA NEC	2452	CHR LYMPHOCYT THYROIDIT
71659	POLYARTHRITIS NOS-MULT	2463	HEMORR/INFARC THYROID
72211	THORACIC DISC DISPLACMNT	25061	DIAB NEURO MANIF JUVEN
7248	OTHER BACK SYMPTOMS	2754	DIS CALCIUM METABOLISM
78053	HYPERSOMNI W SLEEP APNEA	2859	ANEMIA NOS
78057	OTH & UNSP SLEEP APNEA	4010	MALIGNANT HYPERTENSION
7862	COUGH	40391	HYPER RENAL DIS W/FAIL
7880	RENAL COLIC	41181	CORONARY OCCLUSN W/O MI
8020	NASAL BONE FX-CLOSED	4370	CEREBRAL ATHEROSCLEROSIS
80701	FRACTURE ONE RIB-CLOSED	4549	VARICOSE VEIN OF LEG NOS
80702	FRACTURE TWO RIBS-CLOSED	4555	EXT HEMRRHOID W COMP NEC
9640	POISONING-IRON/COMPOUNDS	4557	THROMBOS HEMORRHOIDS NOS
9670	POISONING-BARBITURATES	53510	ATR GASTRI W/O HEMORRHAG
9698	POISON-PSYCHOTROPIC NEC	541	APPENDICITIS NOS
9770	POISONING-DIETETICS	55011	RECUR UNIL ING HERN-OBST
9948	EFFECTS ELECTRIC CURRENT	55090	UNILAT INGUINAL HERNIA
9975	SURG COMPL-URINARY TRACT	55093	RECUR BILAT INGUIN HERN
9988	SURGICAL COMPLICAT NEC	55301	RECUR UNIL FEMORAL HERN
00841	STAPHYLOCOCC ENTERITIS	55329	VENTRAL HERNIA NEC
25061	DIAB NEURO MANIF JUVEN	57420	CHOLELITHIASIS NOS
34510	GEN CONVUL EPIL W/O INTR	5758	DIS OF GALLBLADDER NEC
3462	VARIANTS OF MIGRAINE	585	CHRONIC RENAL FAILURE
59389	RENAL URETERAL DIS NEC	6259	FEM GENITAL SYMPTOMS NOS
7806	PYREXIA UNKNOWN ORIGIN	V581	MAINTENANCE CHEMOTHERAPY
7807	MALAISE AND FATIGUE	V725	RADIOLOGICAL EXAM NEC

Figure 1-1. (Continued)

Code	Diagnosis	Code	Diagnosis
68110	CELLULITIS. TOE NOS	71594	OSTEOARTHROS NOS-HAND
6850	PILONIDAL CYST W ABSCESS	71613	TRAUM ARTHROPATH-FOREARM
7283	MUSCLE DISORDERS NEC	71789	INT DERANGEMENT KNEE NEC
7503	CONG ESOPH FISTULA/ATRES	71841	JT CONTRACTURE-SHLDER
7510	MECKEL'S DIVERTICULUM	71886	JT DERANGEMENT NEC-L/LEG
7842	SWELLING IN HEAD/NECK	71925	VILLONOD SYNOVIT-PELVIS
7856	ENLARGEMENT LYMPH NODES	7271	BUNION
8024	FX MALAR/MAXILLARY-CLOSE	72751	POPLITEAL SYNOVIAL CYST
85402	BRAIN INJ NEC-BRIEF COMA	73023	OSTEOMYELIT NOS-FOREARM
86800	INTRA-ABDOM INJ NOS-CLOS	7322	FEMORAL EPIPHYSIOLYSIS
8730	OPEN WOUND OF SCALP	73391	ARREST OF BONE GROWTH
9110	ABRASION TRUNK	73399	BONE CARTILAGE DIS NEC
9222	CONTUSION ABDOMINAL WALL	73642	GENU VARUM
9895	TOXIC EFFECT VENOM	73689	OTH ACQ LIMB DEFORMITY
035	ERYSIPELAS	80843	PELV FX-CLOS/PELV DISRUP
1649	MAL NEO MEDIASTINUM NOS	81240	FX LOWER HUMERUS NOS-CL
42781	SINOATRIAL NODE DYSFUNCT	81241	SUPRCONDYL FX HUMERUS-CL
72981	SWELLING OF LIMB	81301	FX OLECRAN PROC ULNA-CL
73320	CYST OF BONE NOS	81383	FX RADIUS W ULNA NOS-CL
78650	CHEST PAIN NOS	81401	FX NAVICULAR. WRIST-CLOS
99601	MALFUNC CARDIAC PACEMAKE	81500	FX METACARPAL NOS-CLOSED
7840	HEADACHE	8245	FX BIMALLEOLAR-OPEN
1420	MALIG NEO PAROTID	82534	FX CUNEIFORM. FOOT-OPEN
4618	OTHER ACUTE SINUSITIS	83101	ANT DISLOC HUMERUS-CLOSE
462	ACUTE PHARYNGITIS	83300	DISLOC WRIST NOS-CLOSED
4660	ACUTE BRONCHITIS	83309	DISLOC WRIST NEC-CLOSED
4739	CHRONIC SINUSITIS NOS	8360	TEAR MED MENISC KNEE-CUR
475	PERITONSILLAR ABSCESS	8400	SPRAIN ACROMIOCLAVICULAR
75027	DIVERTICULUM OF PHARYNX	84201	SPRAIN CARPAL
7806	PYREXIA UNKNOWN ORIGIN	8822	OPEN WOUND HAND W
2396	BRAIN NEOPLASM NOS		TENDON
3501	TRIGEMINAL NEURALGIA	8911	OPEN WND KNEE/LEG-COMPL
3558	MONONEURITIS LEG NOS	1725	MALIG MELANOMA TRUNK
45989	CIRCULATORY DISEASE NEC	1730	MALIG NEO SKIN LIP
72252	LUMB/LUMBOSAC DISC DEGEN	1733	MAL NEO SKIN FACE NEC
7802	SYNCOPE AND COLLAPSE	6111	HYPERTROPHY OF BREAST
8460	SPRAIN LUMBOSACRAL	V501	PLASTIC SURGERY NEC
8500	CONCUSSION W/O COMA	74900	CLEFT PALATE NOS
8501	CONCUSSION-BRIEF COMA	74904	BILAT CLEFT PALATE-INC
85400	BRAIN INJURY NEC	74924	BILAT CLFT PALAT/LIP-INC
9529	SPINAL CORD INJURY NOS	75029	PHARYNGEAL ANOMALY NEC
9961	MALFUNC VASC DEVICE/GRAF	8026	FX ORBITAL FLOOR-CLOSED
1178	DEMATIACIOUS FUNGI INF	87353	OPEN WOUND LIP-COMPLICAT
3542	ULNAR NERVE LESION	94420	2ND DEG BURN HAND NOS
V540	REMOVAL INT FIXATION DEV	99679	OTH COMP INT PROSTH DEV
7092	SCAR FIBROSIS OF SKIN	9981	HEMORR COMPLIC PROCEDURE
71102	PYOGEN ARTHRITIS-UP/ARM	5240	MAJOR ANOM OF JAW SIZE
71430	JUV RHEUM ARTHRITIS NOS	52410	UNSPEC JAW-CRANIAL ANOMA

(Continued on next page)

Figure 1-1. (Continued)

Code	Diagnosis	Code	Diagnosis
52469	OTH SPE TEMP JOINT DISOR	64683	PREG COMPL NEC-ANTEPART
5249	DENTOFACIAL ANOMALY NOS	64893	OTH CURR COND-ANTEPARTUM
73028	OSTEOMYELIT NOS-OTH SITE	65103	TWIN PREGNANCY-ANTEPART
80221	FX CONDYL PROC MANDIB-CL	8470	SPRAIN OF NECK
80222	SUBCONDYLAR FX MANDIB-CL	76	OB, NOT DEL
80230	MANDIBLE FX NOS-OPEN	64403	THRT PREM LABOR-ANTEPART
61	ORAL SURGERY	64501	PROLONGED PREG-DELIVERED
1881	MAL NEO BLADDER-DOME	64661	GU INFECTION-DELIVERED
2220	BENIGN NEOPLASM TESTIS	64721	OTHER VD-DELIVERED
2765	HYPOVOLEMIA	64801	DIABETES-DELIVERED
5951	CHR INTERSTIT CYSTITIS	64821	ANEMIA-DELIVERED
5989	URETHRAL STRICTURE NOS	64831	DRUG DEPENDENCE-DELIVER
5992	URETHRAL DIVERTICULUM	64881	ABN GLUCOSE TOLER-DELIV
6011	CHRONIC PROSTATITIS	64883	ABN GLUCOSE-ANTEPARTUM
6082	TORSION OF TESTIS	650	NORMAL DELIVERY
V556	ATTEN TO URINOSTOMY NEC	65281	MALPOSITION NEC-DELIVER
V670	SURGERY FOLLOW-UP	65291	MALPOSITION NOS-DELIVER
7530	RENAL AGENESIS	65451	CERVICAL INCOMPET-DELIV
7536	CONGEN URETHRAL STENOSIS	65611	RH ISOIMMUNIZAT-DELIVER
7880	RENAL COLIC	65630	FETAL DISTRESS-UNSPEC
99659	MALFUNC OTH DEVICE/GRAFT	65641	INTRAUTER DEATH-DELIVER
99665	INF GENITOURINARY DEVICE	65821	PROLONG RUPT MEMB-DELIV
99669	INF OTH INTERNAL PROSTH	66021	ABN PELV TIS OBSTR-DEL
2199	BENIGN NEO UTERUS NOS	66041	SHOULDER DYSTOCIA-DELIV
2333	CA IN SITU FEM GEN NEC	66131	PRECIPITATE LABOR-DELIV
2363	UNC BEHAV NEO FEMALE NEC	66191	ABNORMAL LABOR NOS-DELIV
2851	AC POSTHEMORRHAG ANEMIA	66221	PROLONG 2ND STAGE-DELIV
5990	URIN TRACT INFECTION NOS	66311	CORD AROUND NECK-DELIVER
6238	NONINFLAM DIS VAGINA NEC	66401	DEL W 1 DEG LACERAT-DEL
6289	FEMALE INFERTILITY NOS	66410	DEL W 2 DEG LACERAT-UNSP
64883	ABN GLUCOSE-ANTEPARTUM	66411	DEL W 2 DEG LACERAT-DEL
7890	ABDOMINAL PAIN	66420	DEL W 3 DEG LACERAT-UNSP
9988	SURGICAL COMPLICAT NEC	66421	DEL W 3 DEG LACERAT-DEL
57450	CHOLEDOCHOLITHIASIS NOS	66441	OB PERINEAL LAC NOS-DEL
5921	CALCULUS OF URETER	66540	HIGH VAGINAL LACER-UNSP
64233	TRANS HYPERTEN-ANTEPART	66541	HIGH VAGINAL LACER-DELIV
64243	MILD/NOS PREECLAMP-ANTEP	66551	OB INJ PELV ORG NEC-DEL
64273	TOX W OLD HYPER-ANTEPART	66951	FORCEP DELIV NOS-DELIVER
64293	HYPERTENS NOS-ANTEPARTUM	64254	SEV PREECLAMP-POSTPARTUM
64323	LATE VOMIT PREG-ANTEPART	64664	GU INFECTION-POSTPARTUM
64403	THRT PREM LABOR-ANTEPART	V3000	SING.LIVEBORN,HOSP,W/O C

Source: Ambulatory Care Advisory Group, Inc.

As a planning strategy to meet the growing need for the case management of short-stay discharges, providers must quantify the level of one-, two-, and three-day LOS by diagnosis, program, and service. Operational issues of initial processing, staging, treatment/service, recovery, and ultimate disposition should be assessed and responsive procedures implemented to adequately prepare for these patients. Also, physical space and program configurations will need to be evaluated in tandem, given that most facilities have not proactively planned for changing operations to serve a changing patient population. Finally, providers also can expect that, at some point in the future under managed care directives, some patients in short-stay care programs might require expedited discharge to further reduce the costs of care. In these instances, hospitals might do well to affiliate with home care programs or other alternative providers.

• Conclusion

Outpatient care will emerge as a key focal point of health care reform efforts because it represents an alternative to inpatient hospitalization. Although hospitals have long provided outpatient services, organizing and delivering these services has become increasingly complicated. To this end, many health care organizations are applying traditional case management approaches to increase the efficiency of the outpatient care process.

References

1. Anderson, H. Are hospitals ready for more growth in ambulatory care? *Hospitals* 65(12):34–35, June 20, 1991.

2. Big companies see health costs slowing. *Wall Street Journal,* Oct. 22, 1993, p. A2.

3. McMurray, S. DuPont to cut health care benefits in '94. *Wall Street Journal,* Jan. 5, 1993, p. A3.

4. Ruffenach, G. Firms use financial incentives to make employees seek lower health care fees. *Wall Street Journal,* Feb. 9, 1993, p. B1.

5. Kenkel, P. Illinois Blues will require specialists to follow clinical practice rules. *Modern Healthcare* 23(46):70, Nov. 15, 1993.

6. Felsenthal, E. Maine limits liability for doctors who meet treatment guidelines. *Wall Street Journal,* May 3, 1993, p. 1.

7. Anders, G. Massachusetts Blue Cross's expected cut in infusion costs shows insurers' clout. *Wall Street Journal,* Nov. 2, 1993, p. A3.

8. Lutz, S. Discount cataract project starts. *Modern Healthcare* 23(17):22, Apr. 26, 1993.

9. Burns, J. Stocks slide as patient volume, prices fall. *Modern Healthcare* 23(18):16, May 3, 1993.

10. Burns.

11. Winslow, R. Health-care providers try industrial tactics to reduce their costs. *Wall Street Journal,* Nov. 3, 1993, p. 1.

12. Milliman & Robertson: 24 percent of admissions unnecessary. *Health Care Strategic Management* 10(2):6, Feb. 1992.

13. Primary care clinics will score points for cost, quality, access goals. *Hospitals & Health Networks* 67(22):31, Nov. 20, 1993.

14. Kenkel, P. Mayo Clinic strengthens ties with Deere. *Modern Healthcare* 23(1):17, Jan. 4, 1993.

15. Burda, D. Study—mergers cut costs, services, increase profits. *Modern Healthcare* 23(46):4, Nov. 15, 1993.

16. Taravella, S. Southern California merger to form "Medical Supergroup." *Modern Healthcare* 23(36):12, Sept. 7, 1993.

17. De Lafuente, D. Doctors' orders: integrate. *Modern Healthcare* 23(18):25–26, 31–32, May 3, 1993.

18. De Lafuente, p. 32.

19. Burda, D. Lahey Clinic leads charge in battle for primary-care turf. *Modern Healthcare* 23(17):34, Apr. 26, 1993.

20. Matson, T. Ambulatory care to drive hospital services in 1990's. *Health Care Strategic Management* 9(3):16–18, Mar. 1991.

21. Matson, T. Deployment of outpatient technologies: the hospital-based versus freestanding dilemma. *Administrative Radiology* 10(9):30–33, Sept. 1991.

22. Matson, Deployment of outpatient technologies, p. 30.

23. Matson, T. *Restructuring for Ambulatory Care: A Guide to Reorganization.* Chicago: American Hospital Publishing, 1990, p. 123.

24. Matson, Ambulatory care to drive hospital services in 1990's.

Chapter 2

Introduction to Outpatient Case Management

Michelle Regan Donovan

• Introduction

These are trying times for the health care community. As our elected leaders champion bold initiatives to improve access to care, enhance quality, and reduce costs, the country braces itself for the aftershocks. It is, after all, the providers, payers, practitioners, and patients who ultimately must make the restructured delivery system work.

But in preparing the way for true reform, perhaps the nation is already reaping its greatest potential benefits. The collaboration of health care organizations and insurance companies, affiliations among professional disciplines, and the sharing of business and community resources, unthinkable just a few years ago, reflect a new reality and the embryonic transformation of the health care industry. These integrated systems and allied enterprises are the first steps toward establishing organized care delivery systems that embrace the quality controls, economic savings, and practical payment mechanisms that it has long been hoped would supersede today's complex and fragmented health care system.

In seeking to realize the nation's medical and social ideals, policymakers, insurers, businesses, and health care providers have come to rely heavily on a host of local networks and initiatives generically labeled "case management." Unfortunately, understanding these case management programs—their origins and their many promising applications in contemporary practice—and how to develop them has lagged behind the rapid shift to outpatient sites and services. Case management offers the health care industry and its consumers a multitude of program models and as many definitions of practice and function. However, the framework, applications, and ultimate goals for each model are uncommonly similar. In a global context, the practice of case management relates to a variety of approaches for planning, providing, coordinating, and financing health care across a broad service continuum. Under the auspices of health and human services, *case management* is best defined as a dynamic strategy for organizing services across provider lines, between people and systems, to effect optimal client outcomes, achieve continuity and quality of care, and reduce cost.

Case management is a sound strategy for a new era of health care delivery. It is at once an elegantly simple concept that has stood the test of time and a revolutionary force that is shaping the health care delivery system of tomorrow. Expanding on provider-driven programs that target a diverse array of community and consumer needs, case management today must focus on the ambulatory care arena, especially the growing population of subacute patients. The time is ripe for programs that can link providers, practitioners, payers, patients, and families together in an ever-expanding continuum of care.

This chapter defines case management and explains how it has come to be used with outpatient populations. It also identifies the general categories of case management applications in health care today and discusses the trends that signal the growth of outpatient case management in the future.

• Case Management Defined

Any organized program that coordinates individual patient care throughout the entire continuum of services and settings might qualify as case management. By assigning expert managers to follow individual clients and guide them through the most appropriate course of interventions and referrals, case management aspires to meet the client's specific and changing needs in the most efficient manner possible.

Various health care and professional organizations have already demonstrated the practical application of case management principles in hospital inpatient as well as home health settings. In the wake of the recent clamor for public and payer policies to limit staggering hospital costs, case management has become a veritable growth industry. Carefully implemented and properly run inpatient case management programs can enhance quality, lower costs, and reduce length of stay, while achieving both policy and programmatic goals. But it is essential to realize that coordination of care nowadays must extend well beyond familiar hospital bounds to embrace a more comprehensive and integrated perspective for serving an expanding population in an increasingly complex continuum.

• Thumbnail History of Outpatient Case Management

Over the past decade, increasingly sophisticated technologies, new pharmaceuticals, and financial incentives have shifted many procedures from the expensive inpatient setting to less costly outpatient or home care settings. Thousands of acute care beds and hundreds of hospitals have been lost to steadily declining inpatient days and the aggressive shift from acute to ambulatory care. Providers and practitioners in both inpatient and outpatient settings have restructured their delivery mechanisms and practice patterns to adapt to this rapidly changing environment.

Beginning with the sweeping legislation that established Medicare's diagnosis-related groups (DRGs) and propagated by shifting reimbursement trends among other payers, new regulations soon were drafted to spell out acute care admission eligibility, diagnosis-related lengths of stay (LOS), and appropriate settings for specific procedures and levels of care. Professional review organizations were set up regionally, under the Health Care Financing Administration (HCFA), to monitor hospital and practitioner compliance with these newly mandated criteria.

Hospital and insurance company initiatives patterned after these federal efforts likewise aspired to control escalating expenditures by improving utilization and resource monitors. Espousing the concept of individualized patient care management, these private sector endeavors rallied under the banner of "case management." Boxes began to sprout on health care organization charts for new positions of discharge planner, care coordinator, and case manager. Hospital-based home care departments multiplied. And utilization review departments were renamed case management or utilization management to more appropriately reflect their function.

These initiatives, combined with legislative directives and medical practice changes, created a new patient subset in the outpatient care arena. The *subacute patient,* formerly cared for in the acute care setting, could now receive appropriate care in the home or in various short-stay, day-care, or skilled care environments. This growing outpatient category—frequently comprising the elderly, the disabled, the debilitated, or the mentally impaired—requires substantive medical services, transportation, pharmaceuticals, or sophisticated technology outside the traditional system. Further, industry response promulgated a mushroom of innovative outpatient programs—ambulatory and same-day surgery units, diagnostic imaging centers, cancer treatment centers, short-stay observation units, and partial hospitalization arrangements for behavioral medicine—offering more palatable solutions for both patients and insurers, while generating still more subacute patient volumes for the outpatient sector.

Thus, whether subjected to early discharge under the DRG system, denied hospital admission for failure to meet acute care criteria, or simply requiring postprocedural recovery, more and more patients and their families sought access to optimal health care through a wide variety of outpatient resources. Outpatient case management grew with the need to coordinate these clients' movements, ensure their proper care with appropriate resource allocation, and control costs.

• The Climate for Outpatient Case Management

The future holds even greater challenges. If the DRG system is any indicator of what providers might face with enactment of an outpatient prospective payment system, health care providers should be scrambling to prepare for a new reality. Astute planners will be closely watching several key trends:

- The continued advance of outpatient diagnostic and therapeutic modalities, coupled with federal and state reforms, guarantees explosive growth in all ambulatory care services.
- Specialized programs and long overlooked pieces of the overall health care puzzle, such as home health care, portable technology, home infusion therapies, and intensive day-care programs, are enjoying renewed popularity.
- An aging population is demanding services to meet chronic needs rather than the acute care favored in the current delivery system.
- Minimally invasive surgery has sparked a bona fide revolution in ambulatory surgery.
- New technology and progress in AIDS and cancer therapies offer hope of additional outpatient applications.
- Outpatient rehabilitation, infusion therapies, pain management, cardiology, adult day care, hospice, and respite care promise to be among the fastest-growing outpatient market segments.

Case management is quickly emerging as the master link in the chain of services and programs that must be developed to answer these trends. Innovative, well-organized, efficient, and integrated care delivery systems will be paramount to organizational viability in this new reality, especially with outpatient prospective payment looming on the horizon. More important, these systems must emphasize a consumer focus to assist clients and families in accessing and navigating an increasingly complex delivery system.

Currently, there is tremendous momentum for development of outpatient case management paradigms — and with justifiable cause. Progressive hospitals, freestanding care centers, insurers, and communities are beginning to recognize the increasing acuity and diverse needs of their outpatient clients, especially the elderly and the disabled. Many are realigning their missions, visions, values, and organizational structures to better address the special needs of elderly outpatients — the fastest-growing segment of today's marketplace. Regardless of their point of care or access, elderly patients tend to have more problems, such as multiple or chronic diseases or symptoms clouded by myriad drugs or deteriorating mental status. Besides physical or mental disability provoked by illness, this client group also is most likely to experience visual, auditory, perceptual, and ambulation deficiencies, erecting further obstacles to system accessibility and care coordination.[1]

Case management will be featured prominently in the restructured delivery system. In bridging patients and their families to the care continuum, fulfilling a great need for patient advocacy, and improving quality of care and patient satisfaction while reaping cost savings, case management boasts enough features to appeal to any health care constituency.

The Outpatient Arena

There is no doubt that health care reform will be played out in the outpatient arena. Outpatients already outnumber inpatients 10 to 1. Thirty-one million patients were discharged from the United States' more than 5,000 hospitals in 1991, whereas 325 million outpatient encounters, excluding physician visits, were recorded. Most of these outpatient encounters involved diagnostics, procedures, or definitive care as therapy for an acute or chronic medical condition, though some visits were more for prevention or screening. Some necessitated a single unscheduled visit, whereas many others required painstakingly scheduled multiple appointments or preadmission tests as precursors to invasive procedures or acute care admissions. Many outpatients, especially in the subacute category, required repeated visits or extended postprocedural stays, whereas unfortunate others experienced unplanned admission for maloccurrence, complications, or failed discharge planning intentions.

Few of these outpatients — and here lies the problem — accessed a coordinated system that addressed their prescriptive needs with a single call or consolidated services. Many were required to visit multiple points of service on a large medical campus. Others were required to access entirely separate and sometimes remote facilities or campuses. The difficulty of wayfinding on a large medical campus and between remote facilities — a maze for most clients — is especially pronounced for the elderly and the disabled.

Compounding the difficulty of accessing and navigating campus systems is the vexing challenge of matching client needs with services in the expanded, scattered continuum of care. Normally, when an acute care patient is discharged from the hospital, discharge planners and care coordinators arrange the appropriate resources for safe discharge and aftercare. Depending on the level of care required, the patient and his or her family may be referred to home care, social services, physician providers, Meals-on-Wheels, and so on. Having contracted the required services, the hospital discharge planner's or care coordinator's obligation to the patient ends.

For home health care or social services, the patient is assigned an agency-based case manager who evaluates current health care status and recommends medically appropriate alternatives for the coordination of physician-prescribed care. Case management does *not* prescribe medical care or replace discharge planning. Service is discontinued when the case manager or interdisciplinary group decides the patient no longer requires the designated service or when the patient advances to another level in the care continuum, such as the hospital or a skilled care or rehabilitation facility. The patient may then be assigned to a second case manager aligned with the alternate level of care.

Comprehensive care appears rather easily managed when a client is referred from an acute care setting to an outpatient site. However, accessing services or coordinating referrals between outpatient providers poses some daunting challenges. The sheer magnitude and diversity of the ambulatory setting makes it especially difficult to establish a network of appropriate and convenient services tailored for patients' specific needs. Compounding the problem is a distinct lack of supportive information systems for appointment scheduling, information relays, results reporting, and medical record-keeping for outcome and utilization statistics.

A glut of payment plans and reimbursement initiatives creates additional dilemmas in patient processing and care eligibility. Contractual relationships with participating providers designate the vendors or care delivery systems for certain services. With fewer choices come fewer avenues of recourse should there be any miscommunication or scheduling hassles. Patients requiring appointments with multiple providers, clinics, or diagnostics soon find themselves entangled in red tape.

The Health Care Economy

The U.S. economy is divided by the federal government into two sectors: goods-producing and service-producing. Of all the service-producing industries, health care commands the spotlight in federal and state legislatures, as well as among consumers and private industry. Figure 2-1 shows HCFA's account of America's runaway health care spending from 1970 to 1991. Health care currently devours $890 billion annually, currently rising at a 10 to 12 percent rate annually and representing over 14 percent of the U.S. gross national product (GNP). No other country in the world supports such health care costs. All but Canada, at 9.6 percent, spend less than 9 percent of their GNP on health care.[2]

Rising health care costs in the U.S. stem from three chief trends. They are:

1. The nation's changing demographics, featuring greater longevity and the burgeoning growth of an aging and elderly population
2. The progressive role of expensive technologies in diagnostic and therapeutic applications
3. An increasingly educated, guarded, and litigious public

Added to these are the growing numbers of citizens and immigrants who are uninsured, have no access to primary health care, or live in areas where providers are scarce. Often these people seek care for their episodic and chronic health care needs at the only point of care accessible to them—the hospital emergency department (ED). Of all the gateways into our health care system, the ED is the costliest and, for many patients, the least appropriate.

Figure 2-1.   Health Care Spending in the U.S., 1970–1991

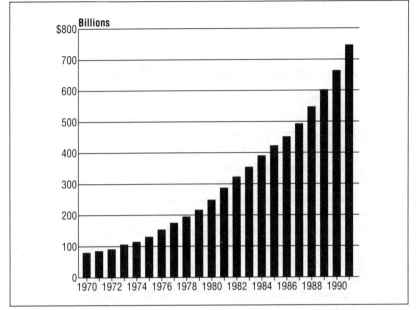

Source: U.S. Health Care Financing Administration.

The Changing Social Structure

Health care reform is not merely an economic movement, it also is a thoroughgoing reexamination of our society and culture. Reform will have a profound and resonant effect, especially on business communities and legal and educational systems. The country must come to grips with the broader social, economic, environmental, behavioral, and cultural forces at work in its health care system, as well as the ethical dilemmas around every corner. Can reality-based reform strike out in a new direction toward "managing health" (that is, preventive medicine), recognizing that ignorance, self-indulgence, addiction, and substandard life-styles are ultimate and major contributors to health care costs? How long can Americans continue to spend and justify the majority of health care dollars on a handful of high-risk, high-cost diagnoses whose origins lie in part in the blatant disregard for health or safety? Is the estimated 80 percent of acute health care dollars spent in the last few months of life justifiable? Will the sheer biomass of an aging population fuel ever-higher health care costs no matter what reform brings? Very soon, the health care economy may refuse to yield to even the strongest cost containment initiatives, because the economy and costs were never the problem in the first place.

But these are questions and observations for the longer term. In the interim, federal and local governments, providers, and insurance companies will be championing care delivery systems, standards of care, and payment mechanisms—all under the general rubric "case management"—designed to make the overwhelmingly complex outpatient arena safer, more efficient, and better organized.

• The Contemporary Practice of Case Management

As mentioned previously, case management comprises a multitude of program models and as many definitions of practice and function. However, all case management models share a common goal: to effectively plan, provide, coordinate, and finance health care across a continuum of services.[3] Traditionally, hospital utilization, social services, and case management departments concentrated staff resources on acute care patients, providing few if any outpatient services for physician practices or outpatient consumers. Out-of-hospital case management applications were delegated to home health providers or private brokering firms. However, patient volume, acuity, system complexities, and revenue shifts from the inpatient to outpatient arenas call for a new agenda.

Looking to the success of inpatient nursing case management and critical pathways for inspiration, similar processes in the outpatient arena can achieve both client-oriented goals (what is best for the individual) and system-oriented goals (what is best for the organization/payer) to effect optimal patient care and system productivity. *Critical pathways* define intense, multidisciplined, and coordinated "care maps" for specific episodes of acute illness or high-risk diagnoses. In the inpatient arena, critical pathways have ultimately reduced LOS and controlled costs by more efficiently utilizing acute care resources and facilitating timely, safe succession to the next level of care. To accommodate a wider variety of caregivers and care settings, however, critical pathways in the outpatient arena must include standards of care and outcome-based goals that will apply regardless of practice base, origin of referral, or point of care. To keep the critical pathways open, the outpatient case manager must work with patients, physicians, claims adjusters, discharge planners, home health agencies, social workers, skilled care or rehabilitative facilities, transportation providers, hospices, and private or employer-based entities. Bridging a diverse patient caseload with appropriate systems and providers in this vast continuum of care requires uncommon clinical, management, and fiscal expertise.

Still, despite these complexities, outpatient case management programs share the five basic goals of their inpatient prototypes:[4]

1. Achievement of expected or standardized patient outcomes
2. Shorter LOS
3. More appropriate or reduced utilization of resources
4. Coordination of care in collaborative practice across a continuum of services

5. Close management and evaluation of patient care processes, pathways, and outcomes

The difference lies in the measures of success in meeting these goals. For example, outpatient LOS might be defined in hours for medical oncology or ambulatory surgery but in numbers of visits for home care or chronic care.

Although for the most part its recent appeal has been economic, case management is above all a human endeavor. For example, pediatric case management programs offer in-home care alternatives that yield much more than cost savings; they also significantly improve the quality of life for acutely ill children and their families. Postpartum and neonatal home care allows the family to share the care of mother and newborn. Middle-aged or elder adults with intact support systems similarly benefit from in-home alternatives to institutional care. Case management allows for the selective choice of care environments based on individual client needs, technology requirements, caregiver aptitudes, and resource availability. And case management is the conduit for other essential human service programs in the outpatient arena, such as housing, employment, social services, rehabilitation, mental health, and community services.

Hospitals have long provided unique arrangements and absorbed the costs of less costly care for individual patients without access or payment plans to cover extended therapies. Some have discharged patients to home care with infusion therapy for necessary chemotherapy administration. Others have paid for and provided housing, food, and transportation for patients without other recourse to medical or social services. However, the components of unique and individualized case management programs espouse unfathomable concepts. Flexibility is essential. In an effort to reduce nursing home bed costs, some state plans empowered individual counties to pay for anything a person needs to stay independent (except land, buildings, or institutional care). For example, when an elderly farmer required hospitalization, the program paid for a week of farm labor so that his cows could be milked. Rationale for providing this service at cost to the state allowed the patient to earn a living, pay his taxes as well as his medical bills, and remain independent.

No longer a theoretical concept, case management has demonstrated its potential value to individuals, organizations, the economy, and society at large. Specific, comprehensive models must now be developed for all outpatient services. Every organization in the health care community must prepare itself to provide seamless care delivery for its far-flung clients.

• The Proliferation of Case Management

The plethora of case management applications in health care today can be categorized broadly into ten types. These include:

1. Payer-based
2. Hospital-based
3. Employer-based
4. Area Agencies on Aging (AAA)
5. Home-based care
6. Private-pay/community-based
7. Clinical (focused)
8. Social services
9. Primary care
10. Rehabilitation

Figure 2-2 further divides these 10 categories into their component models, many of which are described in detail in part two of this book. Despite significant differences in patient population, staffing, administration, payment mechanisms, and other program features, all these models share a strong client focus and follow a case management process based on five basic components: assessment, planning, intervention, monitoring, and evaluation. Figure 2-3 (p. 30) places these similarities in a multifunctional framework that applies to any case management program in contemporary practice.

Several models have been instrumental in the proliferation of case management and will be important influences as case management expands into the outpatient arena. Some of these models are discussed in the following subsections.

Payer Models

In the past decade, the payer sector has been the largest growth area of case management. Responding to escalating costs and declining profit margins, the leaders in payer case management have been health maintenance organizations (HMOs), which employ primary physician "gatekeepers" to ensure access, medical management, quality of care, and cost containment. Insurance lingo — terms such as *capitated* and *discounted* — is now the working vocabulary of hospital administrators, physicians, direct contractors, and accounting personnel. Service and delivery contracts among hospitals, physicians, and community service organizations are commonplace, offering real promise for a cooperative health care delivery system that can provide both quality and fiscal controls. The more seasoned plans include preventive medicine and screening programs as cost containment initiatives. Some organizations construct and operate their own service facilities, whereas others simply contract for services. Eventually, new, smaller breeds of managed care organizations evolved to compete with the giants, and managed care enrollment escalated from 6 million in 1976 to over 41.4 million by 1992. Today managed care claims a significant portion of the insured market.[5]

Figure 2-2. Case Management Applications

1. Payer-based case management

   - Managed care payer
   - Private indemnity
   - Social HMO

2. Hospital-based case management

   - Inpatient acute care
     —Discharge planning
   - Outpatient
     —Program-specific: cardiovascular, oncology, perinatal, postpartum/neonatal
     —Patient-specific: pediatrics, geriatrics

3. Employer-based case management

   - Worker's compensation
   - Employee assistance programs

4. Area Agencies on Aging (AAA)

   - Long-term care
   - Community health
   - Care management

5. Home-based care

   - Visiting Nurse Association
   - Private home health care agencies
   - Hospital-based home health care programs
   - Hospice

6. Private-pay/community-based case management

   - Independent practitioners
   - AIDS

7. Clinical case management (focused)

   - Mental health/behavioral medicine
   - Psychiatric

8. Social services

   - Brokering and linkage
   - Comprehensive

9. Primary care

   - Primary care case management
   - Group practice archetypes

10. Rehabilitation case management

    - Bureau of Vocational Rehabilitation
    - Consumer-directed case management/independent living
    - Cognitive rehabilitation/head injury
    - Physical medicine/physiatry

Taking their cue from successful HMOs and federal capitation initiatives, some private, commercial, and worker's compensation insurers took a proactive stance of similar sorts, intensifying efforts at case management from a fiscal perspective. Many of these insurers took case management to hospitals and physicians to target the small percentage of claims accounting for the greatest health care expenditures of their covered employees or individuals. Some indemnity plans, experiencing declines in enrollment and cash reserves, scrambled to introduce case management programs through their subsidiary companies. Other indemnity insurers, in recent strategies to recapture market share and regain financial viability, have organized managed care enterprises under the umbrella of the parent company.

Figure 2-3.   A Multifunctional Framework of Case Management Practice

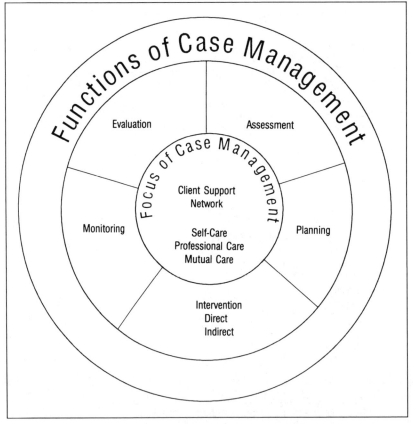

Based on D. Moxley, *The Practice of Case Management.* Newbury Park, CA: Sage Publications, 1989.

Social Health Maintenance Organizations

Social health maintenance organizations (SHMOs) were organized to integrate acute and long-term care settings. The key functions of SHMO case management include determining long-term care benefits/eligibility, prescribing services that integrate postacute and long-term care, closely monitoring clients, and ensuring fiscal accountability for long-term care benefit budgets.[6] The primary advantages of SHMO case management include the availability and rapid linkage of enrolled members to a full spectrum of medical and long-term care services covered by Medicare. These programs are financed on a prepaid, capitation basis by Medicare and by monthly premiums or copays from individuals. Existing SHMO pilot programs at Kaiser-Permanente (Portland, Oregon) and Seniors Plus (Minneapolis, Minnesota) offer extended benefits packages beyond Medicare's skilled nursing home and home health coverage to include intermediate care, in-home nursing services and therapies, homemaker/home health aides, and adult day care. Support services such as medical transportation, emergency response systems, and respite services also are included. The SHMO case management system allows improved and appropriate patient care linkages with all types of resources for a large proportion of elderly and disabled clients whose chronic medical conditions often fluctuate in severity and who require frequent adjustments in types and levels of care. SHMO benefits allow these patient types to be integrated into preexisting practices and medical systems without duplicating the services of other medical and postacute providers.

Community Models

Established community-based case management models, such as home health care agencies, mental health, developmental disabilities, and social service agencies, have grown in size and number with increased patient volumes and a broadened scope of responsibility. Utilization of home health services has risen and become more diversified by client type, as shown in figure 2-4. The number of community hospital home care programs more than tripled from 1980 through 1990, whereas mean annual visit volumes doubled over the same period.[7] The market for home care services expanded to include HMOs, preferred provider organizations (PPOs), employers, physicians, hospitals, insurance companies, nursing agencies, the community, and skilled nursing facilities. Although changing payment incentives and earlier discharges were a primary factor in this growth rate, it was the explosion of sophisticated portable technologies that allowed therapies previously reserved for acute care settings to be provided safely in the patient's home. Subspecialty case management programs for high-risk obstetrical care, infusion therapies, cardiac monitoring, renal dialysis, and assisted ventilation soon followed. Figure 2-5 lists some of the emerging out-of-hospital care

Figure 2-4. User Types of Home Health Agency

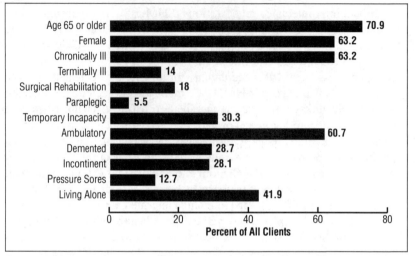

Based on *Users of Home Health Agencies*. (Data from Marion Laboratories *Long-Term Care Digest, Home Health Care Edition*.) Kansas City, MO: Marion Laboratories, 1989.

modalities that have fueled the growth in the home care market. This revolution in out-of-hospital care has yielded significant cost savings for a variety of patient types, as shown in table 2-1.

Primary Care Case Management

The primary care case management (PCCM) model has been enacted by some state legislations (Kentucky, Utah, Michigan, Colorado, and Maryland) in an effort to improve health care access and continuity of care for entitled patients. These often-episodic care seekers usually enter the health care system through the hospital ED, many making frequent return visits, often to a number of local facilities. Obvious patterns of system abuse in duplication of services, diagnostics, treatment, and costs precipitated thorough reviews and strict controls. The fundamental premise of PCCM, cloning the managed care "gatekeeper" concept, is to link Medicaid recipients to physician providers. The PCCM model is intended to render primary and preventive care through a single assigned provider, thus reducing the inappropriate and duplicative use of precious system resources. Keys to the success of PCCM applications include low physician-to-patient ratios, wide geographic distribution, incentive-based payment mechanisms (usually discounted fee-for-service charges), and physician and patient education and behavior modification.

Figure 2-5. Emerging Modalities for Out-of-Hospital Care

Professional Home Care Programs	Infusion Therapies	Home Respiratory Therapies
• Home rehabilitation • Perinatal/Early maternity • Pediatric extended care • Home cardiac and fetal monitoring • High-risk obstetrical care (terbutaline) • Home dialysis	• Hyperalimentation • Intravenous antibiotics • Erythropoietin • Terbutaline • Calcitonin • Immunoglobulin	• Bi-PAP;R (for sleep apnea) • Ventilator

Adapted, with permission, from Ambulatory Advisory Group, Chicago, 1991.

Table 2-1. Cost Savings: Home versus Hospital Treatment

Condition	Cost per Month		Dollars Saved	Home Care as Percentage of Hospital Cost
	Hospital	Home		
Newborn with breathing/feeding problems	$60,900	$20,200	$40,700	33
Cancer chemotherapy	$10,500	$ 3,500	$ 7,000	33
Kidney dialysis	$ 2,000	$ 1,200	$ 800	60
Feeding by tube	$16,600	$ 6,000	$10,600	36
Spinal cord injury	$23,800	$13,900	$ 9,900	58
Disabled cerebral palsy	$ 8,400	$ 4,800	$ 3,600	57

Source: There's no place like home. *US News and World Report* 104:68–70, Jan. 25, 1988.

Area Agencies on Aging

Area Agencies on Aging (AAA), funded under the Older Americans Act, traditionally provided case management and advocacy for low-income and frail elders. But AAAs are expanding beyond their traditional community base to broker the delivery of health care for state entitlement programs and other private factions. The role of AAAs as case managers is controversial, because they are contractors of service rather than direct providers. This model has been criticized for its inclination to "demedicalize" clinical care management for a primarily elder population whose needs are likely dictated by chronic disease, disability, multiple medications or treatments, and frequent physician visits.

• Conclusion

Outpatient case management is one of the country's brightest hopes for health care reform — a thorough restructuring that must proceed at the community level to achieve deep social and cultural change. Every day, escalating volumes of patients are being discharged from acute care institutions into a vast network of home and community programs. The health care industry collectively must address these clients' intense need for coordinated care management and special resources. Outpatient case management programs offer recourse to satisfy the requirements of providers, payers, and patients through skillful assessment of individual health care needs, prudent allocation of available resources, and coordinated care delivery that crosses provider lines to serve an expanding outpatient population with diverse medical, social, and other resource needs.

In anticipation of health reform and system development, the scope and economics of health care must be carefully considered and wisely forecast, with full realization that escalation of costs cannot continue on its current course. In working toward a more equitable system and with empathy for the aging or other debilitated individuals and families outside the confines of the acute care facility and in a fragmented system, it is essential to foster and preserve the stature and tradition of case management. Outpatient case management initiatives are essential to the new reality.

References

1. Donovan, M. R. An endangered resource. *Health Progress,* May 1991, p. 50.

2. Spencer, R. Cutting waste: no cure-all for health care. *The Washington Post,* May 4, 1993, p. A1.

3. Lerman, D., and Linne, E. *Hospital Home Health Care: Strategic Management for Integrated Care Delivery.* Chicago: American Hospital Publishing, 1993, p. 168.

4. Zander, K. Nursing case management: strategic management of cost and quality outcomes. *Journal of Nursing Administration* 28(5):23–30, no date.

5. Spencer.

6. Abrahams, R. The social HMO: case management in an integrated acute and long term care system. *Caring* 9(8):30, Aug. 1990.

7. American Hospital Association. *Meditrends.* Chicago: AHA, 1991.

Bibliography

Abrahams, R. The social HMO: case management in an integrated acute and long term care system. *Caring* 9(8):30, Aug. 1990.

American Hospital Association. *Meditrends.* Chicago: AHA, 1991.

Donovan, M. R. Case management as foundation for home care. In: D. Lerman and E. Linne, editors. *Hospital Home Health Care: Strategic Management for Integrated Care Delivery.* Chicago: American Hospital Publishing, 1993.

Donovan, M. R. An endangered resource. *Health Progress* (Catholic Health Association), May 1991, p. 50.

Feldstein, P., Wickizer, T., and Wheeler, J. Private cost containment: the effects of utilization review programs on health care use and expenditures. *The New England Journal of Medicine* 318(20):1310, May 1988.

Fondiller, S. H. How case management is changing the picture. *American Journal of Nursing* 91(1):63–64, 66, 68, Jan. 1991.

Hafkenschiel, J. Home care past and future. *Health Management Quarterly* 12(3):8, Third Quarter 1990.

Halamandaris, V. The paradox of case management. *Caring* 9(8):4, Aug. 1990.

Hereford, R. Private-pay case management: let the seller beware. *Caring* 9(8):8, Aug. 1990.

Lajeunesse, D. Case management: a primary nursing approach. *Caring* 9(8):13, Aug. 1990.

Matson, T. Ambulatory care to drive hospital services in the 1990s. *Health Care Strategic Management* 9(3):16–18, Mar. 1991.

Matson, T. *Restructuring for Ambulatory Care.* Chicago: American Hospital Publishing, 1990.

Meier, B. Effective? Maybe. Profitable? Clearly. *The New York Times,* Feb. 14, 1993.

Moxley, D. *The Practice of Case Management.* Newbury Park, CA: Sage Publications, 1989.

Petersen, C. AIDS triggers need for early case management. *Managed Healthcare News* 3(7):36, July 1993.

Petersen, C. Pediatric home care: savings plus better healing environment. *Managed Healthcare News* 3(7):38, July 1993.

Physician case management: reimbursement raises a controversy. *Caring* 9(8):50, Aug. 1990.

Pigott, H. E. Psychiatric home health care: one prescription for soaring mental health costs. *Compensation and Benefits Management* 6(4):303, Summer 1990.

Real health care fixes. *U.S. News and World Report,* Aug. 26–Sept. 2, 1991, p. 35.

Smith, J. Trends in psychiatric outpatient services. *Health Systems Review,* July–Aug. 1991, pp. 28, 48.

Zander, K. Nursing Case Management. Presentation for Johns Hopkins Centennial, June 1989.

Zander, K. Nursing case management: strategic management of cost and quality outcomes. *Journal of Nursing Administration* 18(5):23–30, May 1988.

Chapter 3

The Private Payers' Perspective

Steven Sieverts

• Introduction

In various popular magazines and newspapers in 1993, one of America's largest health insurers placed a two-page advertisement that boasted as follows:

> When Lisa was born, her kidneys didn't work. So we helped Lisa's mother learn to care for her. It saved $200,000 in hospital costs. And let Lisa grow up at home.

Referring to the insurance company's "individual case managers," the ad copy went on to say that ". . . they help to find the best available treatment by understanding people's needs and by working with their doctors. In many cases, by discovering alternative methods for treatment, medical costs are reduced. And more importantly, people can recover in a somewhat more comfortable environment. Like home, for instance, with family."[1]

Do insurance plan case managers, as their primary responsibility, really "discover" alternatives that would otherwise not have been chosen? If left on their own, would Lisa's physicians have kept her in the hospital for $200,000 of unnecessary service and deprived her of her mother's loving care at home? And if so, how can a health insurance plan best deal with these problems?

This chapter discusses case management from the private sector payer's perspective. It cannot and does not pretend to speak on behalf of all payers — from commercial insurance companies to health maintenance organizations, from worker's compensation carriers to self-insured large employers — or to represent any more than one person's viewpoint. The purpose of this chapter is to explore how American private health plans might better approach the subject of case management.

• The True Aims of Case Management

Perusal of the recent literature — professional journals, health benefit maga-zine articles and advertisements, industry newsletters — might give the impres-sion that case management is mainly an activity of health care payers.[2-4] Case management often is presented in those media as a payer-conducted program whose sole purpose is to lower the increasingly burdensome costs that health care payers have to bear. Indeed, there is a trade journal primar-ily devoted to case management done by payers.[5]

Case management, however, is, and should be, primarily an activity of community health care providers. Although cost reduction is a hoped-for and likely by-product of case management, a program must do much more than reduce costs if it is to be embraced by patients, their families, and physicians. To be viable in the long run, a case management program must aspire to a higher purpose: to improve the outcomes of care through intelligent management of patients and coordination of the best available resources.

It is truly remarkable that so many people in health care now take it for granted that health insurers have a right — even an obligation — to inter-vene in doctors' and health care institutions' patient care decisions. Those interventions take many forms: requiring prior authorizations if benefits are to be paid for certain kinds of service, imposing denials of payment based on medical records review, and so on.

Care providers and their patients might not always be delighted with what they may perceive as payer interference, but they generally have come to accept the concept that the payer appropriately has authority to influence or even control certain aspects of the payee's patient care behavior. This was not always the case.

• Historical Perspective

Attempts to control health care costs are not unique to the 1990s. This sec-tion leads into discussion of the precursors of health plan case management by tracing the relevant background of health care insurance through the growth of managed care and Medicare.

The Dawn of Health Insurance

When health insurance first began on a wide scale in the U.S., with the found-ing in the 1930s of what came to be community-based not-for-profit Blue Cross plans, the job of the so-called hospital prepayment plans was simply defined. It was to help ordinary wage-earning people obtain otherwise un-affordable hospital care. The plans had two clear aims:

1. To give their subscribers the security of knowing that they could get this costliest of care when needed
2. To assure Depression-squeezed community hospitals of a reliable new source of steady revenues, however modest, to permit continued operations

The Blue Shield physician prepayment plans created in the 1930s and 1940s, as a companion piece to the Blue Cross plans' benefits for inpatient hospital care, had a similarly clear purpose: to help people get costly surgical procedures when needed.

When commercial life and casualty insurance companies later entered the health insurance arena, prompted largely by the opening up of the market during World War II, they had different motivations than the community, hospital, and physician leaders who founded the Blue plans. But in order to compete, the commercial companies adopted essentially the same patterns as the Blues, focusing almost exclusively on paying for the most expensive episodes of care—those involving hospitalizations. Only later did commercial insurance and Blue Cross and Blue Shield benefits expand to cover outpatient care and nonsurgical medical services.

The concept of health insurance was simple. It was no more and no less than a mechanism for people to share collective risk by pooling their funds from employment to pay for needed health care.

Managed Care and Medicare

This simple concept also underlies the creation of what are now called health maintenance organizations (HMOs), which began as far back as pre-World War II as prepaid group practice plans. These plans were not originally conceived to use economic or financial tools to manage how care was delivered. Rather, their function was only to pay autonomous medical groups to provide the services members needed, which was determined by the physicians. Responsibility for "managing" care was left to providers; administrators were hardly involved.

The Medicare Act of 1965 enshrined the same concept into law in the nation's current health insurance program. Like the earlier—but little remembered—temporary wartime program enacted to provide health insurance for the families of military servicemen, Medicare would in no way "interfere" with the practice of medicine, legislators promised. That was no surprise in light of the immense political controversies that preceded passage of the law.

Medicare's design deliberately paralleled the private sector, with Part A covering what the Blue Cross hospital prepayment plans covered, and the separately funded and administered Part B patterned almost exactly on the Blue Shield physician payment plans. The rhetoric that persuaded the

Congress to pass the Medicare Act emphasized the social priority of giving all of America's senior citizens access to the kind of medical care protection that most wage earners, but fewer than half the persons over age 65, had come to expect. If anyone in those days mentioned a role for Medicare and the federal government in influencing how care was to be delivered to elderly people, let alone in actually "managing" their care, it usually was only to oppose so far-fetched an idea.

Even before Medicare became law, however, institutional patterns were evolving that tacitly denied the principle that health insurance existed solely to pay for, rather than influence or alter, the delivery of medical services. In the early 1960s, Blue Cross plans, still linked closely to the American Hospital Association at the national level, originated two major thrusts that were implicitly based on a unique new principle: that health care prepayment should also be a planned force for change in health care delivery to individual patients.

Precursors of Outpatient Case Management

The first new initiative was development of benefits for alternatives to inpatient care, explicitly intended to rein in rapidly increasing hospital costs. The most important of these initiatives covered home health care. The new Blue Cross benefits, beginning in the 1950s in partnerships with key hospitals in New York City and Pittsburgh, were directly responsible for a paradigm shift in home health care. In the wake of this initiative, home health care became something more than the community's altruistic means for delivering public health nursing to the needy chronically ill and to newborn babies and their mothers. Prompted by Blue Cross and the hospitals, home health agencies soon grew to provide a wide range of allied health care services to patients recovering at home—patients who would otherwise have had much longer hospital stays.

The second new health insurance concept conceived by Blue Cross in the early 1960s was dubbed *utilization review.* Most private sector prepayment plans, then as now, paid hospitals for days of inpatient care rather than for inpatient cases or dollars of billed expenses. Because each additional day of care represented a sizeable outlay, health insurers soon established formal review mechanisms to identify and avert unnecessary inpatient stays. Inpatient days were defined as medically unnecessary when care could have been delivered at home or in a long-term care facility rather than in an acute care facility.

Both of these new concepts—benefits for alternatives to acute inpatient care and utilization review—were also quietly built into Medicare's Part A in 1965. By now, they are so well accepted that it may be difficult to recall how radical they seemed at the time.

So the case management concerns of health care payers and providers are not a major departure, new in the 1990s, but rather the logical extension of the seemingly endless effort — going back at least three decades — to bring rising costs under control. The roots of case management are embedded in the principle that to achieve greater cost-effectiveness, payers and providers have to work together to change how patient care is delivered.

• Managed Care as a Payer Activity

The concept of the health insurance plan as simply a payer for care is no longer advocated by any but the most radical conservatives and, implicitly, by some who favor a "single payer" health care system reform. Indeed, by the late 1980s, well ahead of the federal health care reform movement, virtually every major commercial health insurer with a commitment to continue in the business and nearly all of the Blue Cross and Blue Shield plans were acting on strategies to become managed care plans.

As recently as a decade ago, managing care seemed to most observers to be the sole domain of the HMOs. In the early 1970s, HMOs began leveraging their economic and management strengths to shape how their physicians and health care facilities actually provided care to members. Physicians at that time were less than enthusiastic about participating in HMOs that limited their control over patient care decisions, and many physicians continue to exhibit similar resistance to HMOs today.

A wide range of managed care activities, first developed primarily by HMOs, are intended to control costs by limiting the freedom of providers and patients to choose whatever kind and form of medical service they prefer. Such controls include mandating that, unless medically contraindicated, certain surgeries be ambulatory rather than inpatient, or requiring patients' primary care physicians to act as their "gatekeepers" whenever specialty or institutional services might be needed. And, of course, managed care organizations insist that participating physicians refer their patients to participating provider institutions and specialists.

In the 1990s, managed care is no longer synonymous with HMOs. The health benefits marketplace has developed — and is continuing to evolve — various forms of payer–provider contractual relationships, various patterns of benefit plan incentives for patients to get their care in "managed" ways, and various programs that directly involve payers in patient care. Private health insurance that is not grounded in performance-shaping contracts between patients and payers, and between payers and providers, is becoming a rarity.

• The Case Management Unit as a Managed Care Entity

Case management is a managed care activity. For health insurance plans, case management offers a process to influence the care furnished to individual patients in order to maximize benefits while controlling costs. This requires flexibility on the payers' part in interpreting benefits contracts so that, for example, if a plan's standard benefits package does not provide coverage for medical rehabilitation in a low-cost, long-term care facility, the plan's case managers will have authority to approve benefits for such a facility when it is deemed the best available alternative to continued confinement in an acute care setting at a much higher cost. Even more important, payer-based case management demands the close involvement of the plan's personnel in the providers' patient care decisions before and during the time that those decisions are being made. How can a health plan fulfill this role most effectively?

Typically, health plans have established their own case management units, staffed mainly by professional nurses, or, in some cases, have contracted with commercial companies organized to serve carriers. The case management unit's initial assignment is to identify, usually at the point of admission to an acute care hospital or shortly thereafter, patients with diagnoses that carry a high likelihood of prolonged hospitalization and associated high costs. Case managers are then expected to communicate with physicians, patients, and families to help them—or, more precisely, persuade them—to plan lower-cost alternatives to continued acute inpatient care.

What Is the Strength of the Case Management Unit?

The case management unit has three main tools with which to work. The first it shares with any well-run hospital: a knowledge base of the lower-cost alternatives that are reasonably accessible and available for the patients' care. The second is its special contracts with provider institutions that provide care outside the acute care hospital, with the expectation of achieving cost savings. The third is the unit's unique ability to commit the plan to provide benefits for those alternatives, with at least an implied power to withhold reimbursement for continued hospitalization if the less costly options are rejected.

If a health plan is regionally strong—that is to say, if it has a high concentration of enrollment in a geographic community—it enjoys a greater opportunity for success than a plan whose enrollment is widely scattered regionally or nationally. Over time, a locally strong plan can build a roster of lower-cost alternative care providers and, more important, a set of contractual and professional interrelationships with specific home health agencies, ambulatory care facilities, rehabilitation service providers, and so on. These entities will have demonstrated their determination to cooperate with the physicians and hospitals that also contract with the plan—providers that have shown the quality of their care, the reasonableness of their costs, and their willingness to cooperate responsibly. As a strong regional plan's case management unit matures, it gains advantage by augmenting its written provider agreements with invaluable personalized relationships between its case management professionals and the providers of care.[6]

But, as is frequently pointed out, not all high-cost cases should or can be managed effectively in nonhospital settings at lower costs. Some patients are so critically ill that alternatives to acute inpatient care would be clinically inappropriate. More frequent, there are patients whose care could well be provided at home or in an extended care facility but at costs that actually exceed those of keeping the patient hospitalized.[7] For example, for the patient subsisting on parenteral nutrition who needs to have nursing care available around the clock, the community hospital is likely to be the most cost-effective site. As a managed care plan's case management professionals gain experience, they will become more skilled in identifying the cases that offer the best probability of improved care in a nonhospital setting, often with significant cost savings. They also will become more adept at working with the providers who manage the care of those patients.

What Is the Role of the Managed Care Plan?

It is important to remember that HMO and non–HMO-managed care plans (except for the few staff model HMOs) are not patient care providers and therefore do not actually "manage the cases." Physicians and hospitals manage the care of the patients.

The role of the managed care plan is not to usurp the clinicians' decision-making authority and professional responsibility. Choosing therapies, their intensity and focus, the site of care, and the entities that provide care is ultimately the responsibility of physicians working in concert with patients and their families and supported by the hospital's discharge planning group. Despite rhetoric to the contrary, the payer's case managers usually do not take over.[8-9] The health plan's case management unit's job is mainly to achieve cost-saving objectives (hopefully with the patients' best interests in mind) by influencing—directly and indirectly, through education and possibly through incentives—the physicians and others who truly manage the patient's care.[10]

What Should Be the Limits of the Managed Care Plan?

Why should such persuasion be necessary? Why does it seem necessary for payers to intervene if care is to be rendered cost-effectively? Is it true that, if left alone, most physicians will leave a patient hospitalized too long and will not even consider home care or other alternatives? Is it true that, absent outside pressure, hospitals will neglect to plan for posthospitalization services linked to earlier discharge?[11] Is it really true that without payer intervention, care usually will be fragmented, inefficient, and even detrimental to patients?

In its landmark 1989 report on utilization management, the Institute of Medicine indirectly answers these questions:

> The opportunities for savings through high-cost case management by third parties arise from the complexity and fragmentation of the medical care system and the limits built into health benefit plans. Certainly most patients and families with high-cost medical problems start out with relatively little knowledge of what lies ahead of them. . . . Although physicians and hospital staff typically are more informed than patients and families, they too may lack detailed knowledge about the range of options that might benefit specific patients, particularly during the recovery or long-term treatment stages. The care of catastrophically ill patients often involves several specialists, each tending to focus on specific problems, not the whole situation.[12]

However, the difficulty goes beyond many physicians' lack of knowledge about how to employ alternative services and beyond the alleged myopia of some specialists. It also is a product of what patients most deeply expect from their physicians—namely that their welfare should be their physicians' first and foremost concern. That kind of dedication is expected of physicians, and most physicians believe it to be their solemn professional duty. Thus, it is not surprising that the medical subspecialists who attend seriously ill patients prefer to keep them in the hospital where the physicians can pay close attention to what is going on and where nursing and ancillary services are known entities. Likewise, it is not surprising that many psychiatrists prefer to hospitalize patients with mental illness and substance abuse problems and that physiatrists at rehabilitation centers hesitate to send patients back to their communities until full function is nearly restored.

Most physicians are committed to their patients' well-being. Because they want what is best for their patients, quite naturally they want control over the care rendered. They feel compelled to command the dedication of resources to serve their patients, and the hospital—whether acute care, psychiatric, or rehabilitation—is the setting where they can best do that. That compulsion deserves respect, even though it makes physicians resistant to intrusions by people such as health plan case managers, who may sometimes appear to presume to know better what patients need. Indeed, case managers in hospital discharge planning and social work units report similar resistance to their efforts to intervene.

Two common threads run through physicians' complaints about health plan "interference" in their patients' care. They are:

1. Marginal cost considerations ought not to override decisions to provide the best care.
2. A nurse at the other end of a telephone simply cannot know nearly as much about a particular patient's need as the medical care professionals at the patient's bedside.

It would be folly to dismiss these complaints as groundless. Rather, health insurers and managed care plans would be well-advised to ponder the primary purposes of their case management programs. Never mind the boosterism in their ad copy and trade journal articles. If their de facto objective is to alter care to make it less costly, without due regard for what is best for patients, then surely patients, their families, and caregivers alike will respond with skepticism if not hostility. And if case managers insist that their clinical judgment is superior to that of the physicians responsible for the patient's care, they are skating on ice that is indeed very thin — legally, medically, and ethically.

• The Improving Climate for Payer Case Management

Although, given the discussion in the preceding section (that is, the potential for provider–payer antagonism seems inherent in managed care), the climate has been improving. Through two-way education, experience, and cooperation, both parties have come to understand and appreciate each other's responsibility and value in providing patients with high-quality, cost-effective care.

Changing Attitudes

Although many physicians may still prefer to keep sick patients hospitalized longer than may be clinically optimal, and some physicians remain virtually indifferent to the costs of care when their own patients are involved, these attitudes have been changing for a decade or more. The best hospitals have long had active utilization management and discharge planning committees in their medical staff structures. Those committees give direction to nurses and social workers who provide case management for the hospital, and they put major effort into educating attending medical staff. The medical profession's mainstream has internalized the value-laden principles that many seriously ill patients indeed do better at home than in the hospital and that helping to contain costs (for example, by choosing less expensive medications and adapting to treatment protocols) is part and parcel of the imperative to deliver high-quality care.

Moreover, there is growing evidence that case management as a hospital-based function may in fact be more effective than payer-conducted case management. Case management efforts are weakened without full participation of the hospital's medical staff and case managers.[13]

In any event, if a health insurance plan sets out to "manage cases" by presuming that physicians and hospitals are hostile to making care more cost-effective, it will find that prophecy self-fulfilling. Dealing with the physicians and providers as adversaries (and therefore not to be trusted), will guarantee their resistance to the case management program. Dealing with them as responsible professionals who are dedicated to their patients' welfare and offering them assistance and direction in managing cases will almost always win their support.

The Key to Success

The effective case management program, then, does not succeed by "discovering" lower-cost alternatives unknown to doctors and hospitals or just by developing price-advantageous contracts with alternative providers. Rather, the key to its success is its skill in forging strong working relationships, based on mutual respect as well as on well-drawn contracts, with providers. The most productive relationships will recognize and honor providers' primacy in the hierarchy of patient care responsibility.

It is interesting to observe how case management nurses and social workers in high-quality hospitals deal with their counterparts at the local managed care plans. They express professional disdain for health plans that seem to care solely about saving money and whose staffs are both ignorant about the community's resources for posthospital service and indifferent to core values, such as involving the patient and family in care decisions and choosing providers that deliver cost-effective, high-quality services. On the other hand, they express warm professional respect for plans that strive to be helpful and supportive of members of the hospital team, that focus on the individual patient's clinical and social needs, that apply benefits flexibly, and that accept the proposition that, though sizeable cost savings usually can be achieved, saving money is not the primary purpose of case management; patient benefit is.

• Service Contracting with Alternative Providers

For a case management program to succeed in meeting patient care goals and making care more cost-effective, it must deal realistically with the typical community's many providers of "alternative" care—that means learning about those providers, being willing to set and enforce standards, and not being influenced by what appears to be extremely low prices unless quality and integrity are evident as well. It is not unusual, particularly in the metropolitan areas where most Americans reside, for there to be dozens of local home health agencies, home and ambulatory infusion therapy companies, "high-tech" home care providers, outpatient mental health centers, and substance abuse clinics, as well as hospice programs. However, they are not all equal. Many are ethical, humane, professionally competent, and dedicated to providing good, cost-effective care; others are weak in one or more of these areas.

Most patients who transfer from a hospital to the services of one (or more) of these alternative care providers are not overseen by their insurer's case management program. This is as it should be. It is to be expected that a physician caring for AIDS patients, for example, arranges for postdischarge home antibiotic infusion therapies as a matter of routine. Oncologists are expected to transfer terminally ill cancer patients to hospice programs, and psychiatrists to use ambulatory care whenever it seems likely to do the job as well or better than hospital care. Whether or not the hospital's or the plan's case managers are actively involved in these transfers from or substitutes for inpatient care, the managed care plan will properly require its network physicians to refer to alternative care providers with which it contracts.

Provider Selection

Finding suitably qualified providers for contracting can be an arduous process. Dependable criteria — including standards for licensure, accreditation, pricing, and quality of care — are hard to come by.

Providers should be required to be licensed by respected organizations in their fields. If there is a relevant voluntary accreditation program, the providers should conform to its standards even though requiring accreditation may not be feasible. Courts have ruled that it is not acceptable for a payer to refuse to contract with a provider because of a lack of the seal of approval from a private sector third party. Besides, the backlogs at the accreditation agencies, and the required prior years of operation before accreditation, often make it necessary to deal with entities that are unaccredited through no fault of their own. The point is to make sure that unaccredited programs meet the accreditation program standards.

Many states have no licensure requirements for some of these providers, particularly for home and ambulatory infusion therapy providers and for some institutional ambulatory mental health and physical rehabilitation providers. And the very newness of some of these forms of medical service means that there are virtually no useful standards by which to judge many providers' quality of service or prices.

Pricing is an especially difficult problem. High-tech home care, to cite the extreme example, has become a highly profitable business, in no small part because the nonuniform billing practices of the providers frequently make it difficult to figure out exactly what services are being provided. Not only is there a lack of licensure, but there also is no uniformity regarding billing formats, no reliable data on costs, and, in many instances, extraordinarily high prices. It is no surprise that large national health care companies have developed home care product lines and that hundreds and perhaps thousands of small home care businesses have sprung up around the country.

One can only marvel at the ingenuity of some recent entrepreneurs who have built their fortunes on the claim, often with little hard supporting evidence, that their service is less costly than acute hospital care for the same patients. Some such ventures, for example, offer rehabilitation in alternative facilities for persons with major brain damage due to strokes or head injuries. Others offer extended care or subacute care for seriously ill persons requiring hospital-level nursing and ancillary services, taking advantage of a loophole in Medicare's current payment methodology for inpatient care. Some offer outpatient infusion therapy services in nonhospital settings.

Unfortunately, what many of these programs have in common is that their services are not intrinsically less expensive than providing comparable care in otherwise underutilized community hospitals. And there are serious questions about the quality of their clinical and business management in more than a few. In fact, with their leveraged capitalization and high markups, their costs often are higher than other alternatives. And to the extent that some alternative providers may keep patients institutionalized when sensible case management could send them home, their cost-inflating impacts can be significant.

Moreover, unwholesome financial arrangements have a way of springing up where too much money is being made. Late in 1992, the American Medical Association declared it to be unethical for a physician to refer patients to providers in which he or she has an ownership interest, unless there is no other way to find the service. More and more health plans are barring providers from their networks if such conflicts of interest appear. The federal government and some state governments are taking even stricter steps. Indeed, many home care and ambulatory care providers rely on physician owners for their patient referrals. Even without an ownership relationship, it is not uncommon for these companies to pay referring physicians fees for "managing" their patients, presumably with the expectation that those physicians will thereby be induced to make referrals.

With the lack of comprehensive standards, even considering the activity of the accreditation agencies, it is not unusual for alternative providers to practice incomplete and fragmentary patient care recordkeeping, to have few if any requirements as to the qualifications or responsibilities of referring physicians, and to provide little or no medical oversight.

Patients receiving highly specialized services — such as third- and fourth-generation antibiotic infusion therapies, cancer chemotherapies and radiation therapies, and total parenteral nutrition — used to be hospitalized. Maybe they were better off. In hospitals, it can virtually be taken for granted that the physicians are appropriately trained and working within the institutions' medical staff rules and regulations regarding quality of care. The hospital can be relied on to maintain complete, uniform medical records and to work to ensure the competence and thoroughness of the nursing and pharmacy services. Moreover, a crowded hospital environment, with so many health care professionals engaged day and night in collaborative patient care, ensures ongoing peer review.

All of these assurances and safeguards are missing from most home care and ambulatory care providers today. The payer–provider contract must therefore be sensitive to these issues and serve as a safeguard to promote quality of care.

What the Payer-Provider Contract Should Cover

The contracts that a managed care plan executes with home and ambulatory care entities, not only for case management but also for provision of care to plan members, may therefore need to cover ground not typically covered in other provider contracts. The agreements may have to include provisions such as:

- In the absence of mandated standard forms, required conformity with the plan's own billing formats, specifying how certain items — from pharmaceuticals to nursing visits, from medical supplies to medical equipment — are to be listed and counted
- Acceptance of the plan's prospectively established payment allowances for those services as payment in full
- Conformity with the plan's standards regarding medical recordkeeping, professional staffing, continued education, and even such details as drug storage and facility cleanliness
- Conformity with the plan's standards of medical oversight and management of care
- Conformity with the plan's standards for an organized medical staff, ranging from credentialing to quality assurance
- Assurance that physician-owners are not referring patients and that physicians are not being paid (or otherwise rewarded) for referring patients
- Assurance that the provider has the capacity to accept referred patients for service and to provide 24-hour coverage as needed for complications and emergencies

As it happens, some health plans have developed contracts along these lines with local home and ambulatory infusion therapy and high-tech providers, as well as with home health agencies, hospices, and mental health centers. Such contracts should incorporate detailed guidelines and standards, which can be implemented through extensive site visits and team evaluations to select preferred providers based on both quality and cost. This rigorous service contracting procedure also serves to reduce the plan's contracts with regional providers in these categories to a manageable number.

A Case in Point

Blue Cross and Blue Shield of the National Capital Area, serving the Washington DC region, has long employed a highly effective process for selecting the providers with which it contracts for these services. For the most part, the plan's selection process is driven by real differences in the strength of providers' professional staffing, clinical management, medical oversight, and medical records. The selected providers participate in the plan's managed care programs and are used as the primary resources for patients in its case management programs.

The selection process has been a winner for the plan, its members, and its chosen providers alike. The plan's prospectively determined payment rates in high-tech home care, for example, average more than 50 percent below the providers' prices. Research demonstrates that these providers cover their full costs and make a reasonable rate of return even at the plan's reduced payment levels. This is related in part to the higher service volume these arrangements generate, contributing to a lowering of unit costs.

Not surprisingly, hospitals and physicians, as well as the local insurers' case managers, frequently have no idea of the extraordinary inefficiency of many of these providers and how high their profit margins are (excluding, of course, most traditional home health agencies, hospices, and other familiar community-based resources). They also have little understanding of how deficient many of these providers are in maintaining basic levels of integrity and quality in medical care, because they have few benchmarks or standards to apply at the present time. That will surely change in the not-too-distant future.

• Shared Commitment to Change

There is ongoing debate among hospital governing boards, medical staffs, and administrators as to how to manage and accommodate the changing scenario in health care delivery and managed care. The question, though phrased in numerous ways, usually boils down to: How can our hospital survive and thrive when more and more of our patients are members of HMOs and managed care preferred provider organizations (PPOs)?

The answer is quite simple, and the hospital's approach to case management makes a fine illustration. There are only two conceptual alternatives from which to choose:

1. The hospital and its medical staff can deal with the local managed care plans as essentially alien forces, focused solely on saving money in ways detrimental to the providers, and largely indifferent to their members' need for high-quality patient care.
2. The hospital and its medical staff can seek to internalize the concepts of managed care, making responsible cost containment a priority and accepting as fact that managed limitations on individual provider autonomy are both inevitable and desirable in order to protect quality and to control costs responsibly.

To be sure, there are managed care plans whose practices are questionable with respect to quality management, payment, utilization controls, benefit definitions, and holding to contractual commitments. Further, there are plans whose concept of negotiating an agreement with a hospital is to seek victory over an adversary and whose objectives are mainly to pay as little as possible, with little regard for their members' welfare. And there are health plans that, in effect, view hospitals as buildings with facilities and staff to be leased, not as organized medical care institutions responsible for quality, efficiency, and community service. In other words, there may be some health plans whose values are so contrary that hospitals may have appropriate misgivings about entering into contracts with them and cooperating with their case managers.

On the other hand, some hospitals approach contract negotiations armed with tough lawyers and commercially oriented managed care consultants, seeking ways to maximize their market share and revenues, without any apparent willingness to cooperate with health plans in such core undertakings as utilization management, network referrals, and case management. Typically, such hospitals tend to have medical staffs that resist joining managed care plans, just as they resist the institutions' own programs of quality assurance and cost management. Ethically and socially responsible managed care plans may be obliged in the immediacy of marketplace pressures to enter into contracts with some of these hospitals, but a marriage between such hostile partners is doomed to fail.

Over time, it is to be hoped that the community health plans and health care providers that have shared commitments to provide high-quality care in a cost-effective manner will be the winners in this rapidly evolving health services marketplace. Development of sound case management programs is a valid way to test and demonstrate how payers and providers can work together to reach results that both sides desire — and that do the right things for patients.

• Conclusion

The keys to a successful case management partnership are shared values and shared goals. Health plans and providers around the country have all the makings of such a partnership.

What health insurance plans are obliged to emphasize — the imperative to keep costs down — is not antagonistic to the provision of high-quality medical care. What hospitals and physicians are obliged to emphasize — the imperative to provide high-quality care to patients — is not antagonistic to cost management.

Case management provides a significant opportunity for health plans to demonstrate the strength of their commitment to their sickest members' welfare. Additionally, case management provides a significant opportunity for the providers of care to demonstrate that they can ensure clinical quality and humane treatment and at the same time manage costs aggressively.

References and Notes

1. For example, the *New York Times Magazine,* Jan. 17, 1993, pp. 18–19. The same advertisement ran in numerous other popular magazines as well as in trade papers of various kinds during that month.

2. Spitz, B., and Abramson, J. Competition, capitation, and case management. *The Milbank Quarterly* 65(3):348–70, 1987.

3. Davidson, G. B., and others. Modeling the costs of case management in long-term care. *Health Care Financing* 13(1):73–81, Fall 1991. [All five models refer to case management by payers.]

4. Henderson, M. G., and others. A guide to setting up a case management program. *Business and Health,* Mar. 1989, pp. 26–30.

5. *The Case Manager* is published as a quarterly by Systematic Corporation. The numerous advertisements it carries are predominantly placed by health care providers (mainly for-profit) of services ranging from acute inpatient rehabilitation to computerized provider referral registries, and from home infusion therapy companies to nursing homes.

6. LeBrun, P., and Keener, S. B. Case management offers opportunities. *Health Care Strategic Management,* May 1988, pp. 11–12.

7. Gray, B. H., and Field, M. J., editors. *Controlling Costs and Changing Patient Care? The Role of Utilization Management.* Chapter 5. Washington, DC: National Academy Press, 1989.

8. For example, the July/Aug. 1992 issue of *The Case Manager* contains an interview with an insurance company manager of case management services that clearly reflects the view that it is the payer who manages the care being received by patients in case management.

9. The same thrust can be found in: Mazzola, M. Effectiveness of case management: cost savings methodology. *The Case Manager,* Jan. 1991, pp. 56–59.

10. This is the main thrust of the Health Insurance Association of America's 1988 publication *AIDS Case Management: What Health Insurance Companies Are Doing.*

11. That planning by hospitals for earlier discharges and coordinated cost-effective posthospital care is not new, see: Brestow, O., and others. *Discharge Planning for Continuity of Care.* New York City: National League for Nursing, 1975.

12. Gray and Field.

13. Christianson, J. B., and others. Hospital case management: bridging acute and long-term care. *Health Affairs,* Summer 1991, pp. 173–84. This article reports on the mixed results of an Arizona demonstration project in which case management was provided by teams at, but not of, several hospitals. The authors' conclusion is that to be successful, these programs must secure "the cooperation of (hospital) discharge planners and social workers, mobilizing physicians' involvement and support. . . ."

Chapter 4

Outpatient Program Development

David P. Moxley, PhD

• Introduction

Development of an outpatient case management program requires the strong guidance of well-informed planners. Before the development process begins, however, they must thoroughly familiarize themselves with the special needs of the program's target outpatient population and with the case management approaches best suited to serve those needs. Determining how best to design and implement a program will require systematic planning, careful development, and frequent evaluation. Gaining the proper perspective is the first step in a systematic, stepwise development effort.

It is essential that planners acknowledge the value as well as the complexity of such an endeavor in the outpatient arena. It is equally important that they formulate the initial program purpose before proceeding with the more detailed examination and integration of the program's community, organizational, and system components. The programmatic design must reflect the mission, vision, values, and goals of the organization and its professional staff. And fundamental planning objectives should address the community's particular needs, such as social problems, health concerns, and resource availability and accessibility.

Variations in policy mandates, programmatic purposes and functions, models, staffing, and client groups pose a significant challenge for meaningful and effective case management program development. A number of factors must be considered when conceptualizing, designing, developing, and evaluating case management programs in outpatient settings. This chapter highlights these critical variables and the challenges they can create. Case examples are used to depict the role of these critical variables in program development.

• Two Schools of Thought

The ubiquity of case management in health and human services attests to its growing popularity as a means of achieving policy and program goals.

In actual practice, however, policy and program goals may conflict, because there are two schools of thought regarding application of case management principles. One school views case management as a tool to forge a more efficient health care delivery system via care management, gatekeeping, or service rationing. The other school views case management as a better way to represent consumers, patients, and clients by guiding them through what is often a frustrating bureaucracy and communicating their needs to multiple providers.[1]

Is the purpose of case management to create delivery systems that better manage people and the resources they need? Is it to help patients obtain the services, supports, and resources they need or want? Or, does case management reconcile these opposing forces, fulfilling the pressing need for systemwide efficiency and effectiveness while accommodating patients' preferences and desire for equity?[2,3]

Because this emerging field is fraught with such conflicting tendencies, program developers must work to understand and resolve them from the beginning. It is wise, therefore, to establish very early in the process of program development the purpose of case management within the context of outpatient health care.

• Diverse Approaches to Program Development

The manifold purposes of case management have expressed themselves in a variety of diverse approaches to program development, especially in the field of health and human services. These variations are attributable to variations in policy mandates, economic issues, philosophical commitments, social problems and health concerns, professional discipline and socialization, and consumer activism, to name only a few salient factors. Case management programs are being implemented in every corner of the health and human services field: maternal and child health services, aging, developmental disabilities, mental health and psychiatric rehabilitation, head injury rehabilitation, immigration, income maintenance, primary health care, job training, managed health care, and child welfare.[4-14]

To the layperson, the wide variety of case management programs and approaches may appear senseless and duplicative; however, it reflects the growing challenge of offering a broad array of outpatient health and human services within an integrated, cross-system framework that must address the multiple determinants of health, including biological, environmental, social, psychological, and cultural factors.[15] Whether the program is designed to maintain the health of people who are well or at risk, or to help people with disabilities enjoy a decent quality of life, case management is linked to the recognition that health, illness, and disability are best understood within the context of a multivariate and complex model of determinants.[16]

Future delivery systems must respond to this complexity through responsive programmatic arrangements.

Other social, policy, and technological factors have influenced the proliferation of case management. The driving forces include: deinstitutionalization, home-based care, increasing lifespans, the interaction of poor health status with other social problems such as poverty, the reality of serious disability and resulting social dependency, the husbanding of precious resources, and cost control.[17] Another influential driving force is a growing societal commitment to deliver services in smaller, community-based outpatient facilities outside the boundaries of major institutions. The perceived need for case management usually can be linked to some policy mandate that underscores the high worth policymakers place on social intervention at the community level.

Specific models of health and human service case management include clinical case management,[18] rehabilitation case management,[19] brokering forms of case management, and case management systems that address the integration of multiple providers into an interdisciplinary practice matrix.[20] But this list does not exhaust the possibilities. By virtue of its diversity, case management is growing to mean many different things to many different people. It often is seen as a means of connecting people to systems, systems to people, and systems to systems on behalf of clients with multiple, complex, and long-term service and support needs.[21] Suffice it to say, case management is currently seen by many stakeholders in the health care arena as an important and vital programmatic element.

• Initial Considerations for Program Development

An outpatient case management program is shaped in both form and substance by the actual social problem or health concerns the service seeks to address, by policy and administrative mandates and related goals, by stakeholder perspectives, and ultimately by the purpose that guides the case management effort. Program designers must take these factors into consideration and anticipate how they will influence the design of the projected case management initiative.

Social Problems and Related Health Concerns

Often outpatient health services must respond to a population whose social predicaments can cause or exacerbate problematic health conditions. Program planners must be informed about the diverse and multiple needs of the target population and must reflect on how those needs can shape the program's purpose. For example, one urban outpatient health service that targets people who are homeless and coping with mental illness has developed a program that combines physical health services, mental health outreach services, and social services into a complex model of service delivery.[22] To successfully implement an effective and meaningful program, planners had to look well beyond the physical health needs of the target population.

The target population's needs for basic living resources, entitlements, health education, outreach, and ongoing medical management may be striking. Some form of community or regional needs assessment may be required in order to initiate sound program development. To ensure that the case management program will be sensitive to different perspectives, a multimethod approach to needs assessment may be required. Integrating epidemiological analysis, key informant interviews, and the perspectives of potential clients themselves will enable the outpatient health service to consider both the quantitative and qualitative dimensions of case management needs.[23] Consumer perspectives are especially important because consumers may prioritize very practical and essential needs relating to survival and community living over clinical needs that appear to providers to be the most salient and important to fulfill.[24]

Policy and Administrative Mandates

Health and human service programs typically are influenced by a set of policies that mandate their implementation or, at least, strongly encourage their development.[25] Such is the case with case management. For example, Public Law 99-660 identifies the necessity of offering coordinated and integrated service delivery to people with severe and persistent psychiatric problems, whereas Public Law 99-457[26] requires local communities to create interagency structures for the integration of services for young children with developmental challenges and their families, using case management approaches at the client level of service. In conjunction with a needs assessment, outpatient health service administrators and program developers should examine and analyze all relevant policies as well as administrative or regulatory mandates by federal, state, or accreditation bodies.

Of course, other standards can be factored into this initial inquiry. Both the National Association of Social Work[27] and the American Hospital Association[28] have identified standards, functions, and activities for case management services.

Program Goals

Close examination of the policies guiding case management program development, related administrative mandates, and standards promulgated by professional or provider groups, in conjunction with an understanding of the need for case management within a local community, can reveal the goals of the case management program. As noted above, program goals often can conflict in practice, creating tension for consumers, case management staff, and the sponsoring organization.

Following are potential goals of a case management program. These programs may seek to achieve only some of these goals because several of them can conflict in actual practice.

1. To ensure the coordination and integration of services in order to achieve continuity. Often this goal is implemented through individualized health plans involving multiple providers and disciplines that work collaboratively with the consumer and that monitor the delivery of services across service domains and time.[29-31]
2. To monitor the quality of service delivery by examining what is provided, when, and perhaps how.[32]
3. To exercise social control by reaching out to members of high-risk groups whose health status may jeopardize themselves or other members of the community; engage these individuals in a relationship; and monitor them over time, often with the aim of gaining compliance with a medical, service, or behavioral regimen.
4. To offer social support to people who may be isolated, stigmatized, or rejected by significant others because of their health status, behavior, or violation of social norms.[33]
5. To organize instrumental assistance so that people can obtain support to execute the necessary tasks of daily living or have these tasks undertaken for them in the least restrictive setting. Often this goal is achieved by arranging for basic supports such as respite care, homemaker services, home health assistance, mobility assistance, or meal and nutritional care.
6. To engage in cost and resource management so that either cost avoidance, cost-effectiveness, or efficiency is achieved, typically through utilization management, gatekeeping, and prior authorization activities.[34]
7. To serve as an advocate to ensure that clients' needs are identified and fulfilled on a timely basis or that clients' rights are respected and addressed during the course of service delivery.[35]

This list does not nearly exhaust the possibilities, given the diversity and ubiquity of case management services today and in the years ahead. But the diversity of these goals reflects the challenge inherent in packaging case management and achieving a clear sense of its purpose.[36] Case management programs often employ a blend of administrative, management, evaluative, and psychosocial functions organized to address the delivery of services at several levels, including the individual client, the service system, and the general community. The resulting goal mix creates a dilemma: Can the program effectively serve people with multiple, complex, and interacting conditions that require high levels of resource commitment, while trying to perhaps ration the range, volume, and intensity of services these clients require? Case management mirrors the growing controversies in health care surrounding patient dignity, service relevance and sensitivity, cost control, and quality assurance.

Stakeholder Perspectives

Administrators, health and human service disciplines, provider groups, funders, regulators, and clients and their significant others and advocates all have a stake in case management program development. Such pluralism means that each group may expect something different of the case management program, and so each must be involved in shaping the program's focus.

A key decision in getting started is the extent to which such groups should be involved in the planning process. Obtaining their input as part of the needs assessment process will assist program developers in capturing the range of perspectives and expectations of these various audiences.[37] Achieving an understanding of these perspectives may result in a more valid program design and clarity of focus so that funders, case management staff, and clients have a good understanding of what services the program will offer, how it will offer these services, and what ultimately will be achieved. Each of the seven goals listed above suggests something different about the ultimate outcomes of the program. The possibility of a goal mix, tension created by these different goals, and the possibility of goal displacement should be in the front of program developers' minds.[38]

Program planners may wish to consider forming a steering committee for program development. The committee, composed of representatives from all groups with a vested interest, can help shape the program's mission, substance, and function and offer input into the selection and prioritization of goals.

Formulation of an Initial Purpose

The chief product of this phase of program development is an understanding of the initial purpose of the case management program. Formulation of the initial purpose intertwines with other initial program development activities such as data collection, policy analysis, stakeholder involvement, environmental scanning, and reflection on the motivations of the outpatient health service to add a case management component. Understanding the health, human service, and support needs of the intended beneficiaries, as well as other data and policy and administrative mandates, will assist program developers to begin to shape an initial purpose and working mission for case management within the outpatient health service. The relevance of this mission can be further strengthened by considering the input, desires, and expectations of key stakeholder groups and the expectations held by the outpatient health service.

• Understanding the Context of Case Management Service Delivery

The initial working mission of the case management program can be further refined through analysis of its actual context—the specific situation in which the case management program must operate and within which it will be implemented. Three program contexts can be considered:

1. The community in which the program will be operating
2. The health and human service system within which it will be implemented
3. The specific organization that will serve as the host to the program

Community Context

Case management programs are necessarily shaped by the communities within which they operate. Rural and urban settings pose their own distinct challenges for case management program developers, and hold their own distinct strengths and weaknesses.

Rural communities offer certain strengths on which a case management program can capitalize.[39,40] Because people are more likely to know one another in a rural community, the program can tap into case-finding mechanisms, social supports, and community norms that are already strong. Case management programs seeking to incorporate informal support, self-help, and community involvement and action may be able to make use of these rural attributes.

Alternatively, rural communities can create some significant challenges. If transportation systems are underdeveloped, potential clients can easily become isolated. In one rural community, a case management program was struggling along without any system of public transportation. Thus, the program needed to be designed on an outreach basis so that case managers had a lot of physical mobility. Much of case managers' time was invested in driving to clients' homes and assisting them directly with transportation in order to ensure their linkage to needed and appropriate health and human services. The resulting impact on case management productivity is obvious. Without agency automobiles, vans, or other vehicles, case managers had to rely on their own cars and cope with the wear and tear on themselves and their autos.

Many rural communities simply do not have a diverse and elaborate network of health and human service providers. A community hospital, several private practitioners, and perhaps a handful of generalist human service agencies may be all the case management program has to work with. Within this context, implementing a brokering approach to case management—involving the linkage of people to relevant health and human service providers as the principal aim of case management—is very problematic.[41] In addition, achieving interagency coordination of services may be very difficult because of constraints on the availability of providers.[42] In some rural communities, case managers routinely assist clients and family members to migrate from their home communities to urban areas to obtain necessary services and supports.

Finally, some rural communities may have a low tolerance for deviance. Strong negative attitudes toward people with serious health, psychiatric, and behavioral problems may exist and, therefore, clients may be easily stigmatized, labeled as poor candidates for service, or suffer discrimination or outright rejection. In one situation, a client with serious mental illness and a major health problem was "cooled out" by the local hospital and physicians because she was labeled as uncooperative, noncompliant, and childish in her interactions. Health providers withdrew preventive, monitoring, and outreach services, and the client began to postpone treatment until a health crisis forced her to contact emergency medical services. Despite her high utilization of expensive health resources, the attitudes of primary health providers precluded their efforts to manage this case effectively. Although rural health systems certainly have no monopoly on misunderstanding and discrimination, a close-knit community may more readily solidify and reinforce such attitudes.

Urban communities may offer people with potentially stigmatizing problems more anonymity, and tolerance for "differentness," deviance, and alternative life-styles may be higher in urban areas than in rural communities. Urban case management programs also may enjoy stronger service infrastructures composed of an array of public, private, and not-for-profit health and human service providers. And despite severe cutbacks in transportation resources in many urban centers, cities still have public bus systems, connector systems, and paratransit alternatives to support the mobility of clients.

Yet, urban contexts pose other challenges to case management program development. Urban health, mental health, and social service systems often are overloaded by the concentration of potential clients and the staggering complexity of problems these individuals present to urban service delivery systems. Health problems stemming from homelessness, substance abuse, mental illness, or family disorganization are all too common in our nation's cities. Because health problems cannot easily be isolated from other social, psychological, and behavioral conditions in the urban setting, outpatient health services and case management systems must increasingly address needs comprehensively.

Violence and other social control problems may abound in urban centers, and it is not unusual that case managers have to create interfaces between outpatient health services and police departments, court systems, and jails or correction facilities. Often case managers themselves may risk personal safety as assertive outreach approaches dispatch them to homes and neighborhoods in harm's way.

The community context within which the case management program will be embedded must be examined closely. Certainly the salient and hidden strengths of each community must be identified and the contribution of these strengths to the purpose, aims, and implementation of the case management program considered by program developers.[43] In one community, for example, a committed chamber of commerce facilitated collaboration between health and mental health providers and businesses to establish an outreach health program for homeless people in the business loop. Attention also must be paid to structural weaknesses in the community, such as inadequate mental health services or housing and their subsequent impact on how case management functions. Inadequacies in a service system may require the case management program to engage in extraordinary service system development, advocacy, and community organizing efforts.[44-46]

System Context

Case management also may unfold within the context of complex health care systems that have been formed through collaborative agreements, consortia arrangements, or integration of programs or agencies into multiprovider systems. This system context may influence the programmatic configuration of case management.[47] In some health systems, case management programs may be internally driven; in other systems, they may be externally driven; and in still others, a mix of internal and external orientations may occur.

Internal case management may be more oriented toward administrative oversight of service delivery. The case manager may function truly as a "manager of service" with authority to monitor service delivery and identify issues pertaining to utilization, quality, cost, and effectiveness.[48] In this situation, the case manager may act as an internal correction to the system, working with case-level and aggregate data to control service delivery.

Another form of internal case management may involve offering assistance to clients as they move through a complex service delivery system.[49] In this situation, the case manager may ensure that needs of the consumer are identified and that the consumer transverses the necessary services, systems, and departments in a timely manner to fulfill these needs. In one specialized health facility for children with developmental disabilities, a case manager is assigned on initial assessment to ensure that children and families move through the interdisciplinary process in an effective and sensitive manner and that their identified needs are addressed by appropriate disciplines. The case management function culminates in the collation of essential interdisciplinary data, input, and plans, and the case manager helps the family interpret these materials in planning for the next steps in service delivery. The case manager in this sense manages the care pathway, coordinates client movement through this pathway, and troubleshoots any problems, all of which are articulated to achieve service integration.[50] This example also illustrates the importance of assuring clients of a dedicated relationship with at least one professional during the complex course of service delivery.

Case managers also may assume external orientations. Some health systems can comprehensively address the health needs of clients, but there may be entitlement and benefit, social support, and other service needs that the system cannot fulfill. For provision of these external services, the case manager follows along and monitors the status of clients and assures appropriate connections to necessary services, supports, and benefits. The case manager also may follow the client after discharge or between episodes of illness to ensure that linkage and engagement continues, that the client does not become isolated, and that essential needs are addressed and fulfilled. Although case managers in this case may be part of a larger system, they may concentrate their attention on the client's situation in the external community. Under these circumstances, the case manager may be more of an organizer of resources, an ongoing supporter of the client, and a developer of individualized support systems.

Finally, some systems may support independently organized and autonomous case management agencies.[51] One function of such agencies is to comprehensively address the case management of specific target populations without offering any direct health care services. Outpatient health services may interface with such agencies in serving the health needs of certain populations, such as children in the child welfare system, people with developmental disabilities, and people with serious mental illnesses. Program developers may need to identify and review other local case management providers and models to determine whether their outpatient health services pose a problem in terms of mission and purpose, service redundancy and duplication, or other potential conflicts. On the other hand, existing programs might provide opportunities for cooperative efforts.

Organizational Context

The case management program's host organization presents other contextual considerations for program design. Certainly program developers will want to carefully examine the mission, values, and purposes of the host organization to ensure consonance between its culture and the new program in order to ensure acceptance, integration, and utilization.

The disciplinary mix of the host organization is an essential consideration in case management program development. Many health care organizations operate along strict disciplinary lines, with physicians, nurses, social workers, and other health care professionals assigned to distinct roles. Assigning case managers, the desirable credentials of these individuals, and their level of authority are crucial decisions that must be addressed within the discipline orientation of the host.[52] In some settings, for example, physician authority cannot be compromised; case management may be considered solely the domain of the physician, who exercises overall control of every case and allocates specific activities and functions to other disciplines.

Within interdisciplinary settings, however, case management roles may not be allocated on the basis of discipline. Certain core credentials may be important, but the case manager's substantive knowledge of the case, the necessary skills to effectively address the unique needs of individual clients, and the desire to work with specific types of cases or problems are considered the more important qualifications.[53] A range of disciplines may be involved in case management, and there may be considerable flexibility in the assignment of various disciplines to case management functions and activities.

In other settings, professional disciplines may not be a powerful, overriding factor in program development other than to meet accreditation and regulatory standards. Some may even "deprofessionalize" the case management function—and so family members, consumers, and nondegreed staff may all be legitimate case managers. For example, one outpatient program targets its primary health services to Asian immigrants and migrants from Appalachia. Case management is defined as an essential outreach, follow-along, and support function with the express purpose of engaging high-risk clients and maintaining their ongoing involvement in primary health care. The program is staffed by representatives from the target population, who work under the guidance of nurses and social workers.

• Program Design

As planning progresses, case management program developers inevitably will arrive at a point when specific decisions about program design must be made. Initial planning activities give developers an understanding of the needs the case management program will address and the potential purpose it can serve. Understanding the contexts of case management sensitizes program developers to the challenges created by the multiple settings in which the program will operate.

Specific program design decisions will involve formulation of a case management mission, selection of a configuration, and identification of functional case management elements, dosage, and staffing. The cumulative outcome of these efforts is a case management model.

The Case Management Mission

Although case management may have any number of goals, three alternative missions may be considered. These are:

1. An administratively driven mission
2. A mission driven by linkage and support considerations
3. A client-driven mission

An *administratively driven mission* will focus the case management program on the management and control of resources necessary to serve the identified target population. For example, one outpatient program based its mission on preventing duplicative service delivery among people with health problems that were a consequence of both aging and mental illness. The program channeled patients into well-coordinated service structures with unified service plans. Through this means the program sought to reduce the cost of care while still meeting the needs of its service population. A program might pursue this mission when there is concern about gatekeeping, rationing, or cost containment. Interorganizational coordination of services may be a salient feature of such a case management mission in light of economic concerns relating to duplication, overutilization, or inappropriate utilization of service delivery. Of course, such a mission does not preclude concern with ensuring quality and relevance of service, but its primary consideration is system management of the client and ensuring appropriate utilization. Case management often is narrowly conceived in programs with administratively driven missions.

A case management model with a *mission driven by linkage and support considerations*[54] typically is concerned with assessing clients' needs — usually comprehensively — and linking people to necessary services, entitlements, and opportunities. One program serving people with developmental disabilities who are living independently in an urban setting emphasizes linking people to needed mainstream social supports and services. Case management for this program means the management of service linkage and the program measures its performance in terms of whether clients' needs are fulfilled within normalized settings. Such a mission also recognizes the importance of social supports, and so there may be concern about working with families, significant others, and friends to offer enriched supports to clients. A linkage and support mission usually involves multiple providers — perhaps collaborating with primary caregivers — in identifying the broad needs of clients and then organizing, brokering, advocating, monitoring, and evaluating the necessary resources to fulfill those needs. Case management programs pursuing a mission of linkage and support often are broadly focused and concerned with comprehensiveness of service delivery.

A case management program with a *client-driven mission* prioritizes the desires of clients, paying little heed to professionally defined needs.[55] Case management models with such a mission turn on identification of the clients' self-defined needs, and case management service provision is designed to assist and support the client in achieving those self-defined outcomes. One case management program designed to support people with serious health problems in their homes places a lot of emphasis on assessing what people feel they need in order to make daily living with a serious illness possible. The mission of this program is to help people identify their quality of life concerns and then to fulfill these by creating a collaborative relationship between case managers and clients to address these issues. The mission of this program speaks to the fulfillment of client preferences and desires and does not make cost outcomes a focal point of service delivery. Unlike administratively driven case management, client-driven programs are not concerned with outcomes the system desires but, rather, with outcomes identified and prioritized by the consumers themselves. What do clients want? and How do they want to achieve these ends? are the questions that drive this form of case management. Client-driven case management programs incorporate strengths assessments, partisan advocacy by case managers, self-advocacy by clients, creative access to resources through community networks, and ongoing supportive relationships between case managers and clients.[56]

The program mission will flow somewhat naturally from the activities undertaken during program start-up as well as during the efforts invested in understanding the program contexts. But setting aside time to specify a mission is a critical precursor to further programmatic design.

Program Configuration

A case management program can be configured for the provision of service by an individual case manager or by a team of case managers. Many case management programs with a linkage and support mission are configured for individual case managers who maintain their own caseloads of clients and work to link clients to necessary resources. This configuration is effective when clients have specific entitlement and programmatic needs (for example, the need for homemaker services). But clients who have severe disabilities or problems that require ongoing and intensive vigilance may simply need more flexibility and attention than individual case managers can provide.

A team case management configuration is more flexible and responsive for clients whose needs and problems require constant attention to avert the high potentiality of crisis. One variation of this configuration is for a team of case managers to meet regularly (daily or weekly) to share information about clients in their individual caseloads. Team members may then cover for one another during on-call periods such as holidays, weekends, and evenings. This team concept allows individual case managers to expand their potential caseloads without expanding their actual work loads. And when case managers do have to cover for one another, they are better informed and more sensitive to the needs of patients not on their regular case lists.

In another variation of team case management, one team shares the entire caseload and team members in specialized or generalist roles work together to respond to clients' needs. For example, in the Assertive Community Treatment model, which provides intensive case management, clinical, training, and support alternatives for people with serious mental illness who are high service utilizers, a small team of professionals and paraprofessionals work together to maintain their clients in community settings.[57] Team members meet daily to coordinate their objectives, activities, and services.

Regardless of the program configuration, of fundamental importance is ensuring that each client has at least one enduring relationship with a case manager. Case management programs based on linkage and support or client-driven missions recognize the importance of maintaining a dedicated, enduring, and strong relationship between client and case manager. But administratively driven case management programs may underestimate the importance of such relationships and, consequently, discount the necessity of ensuring a good, face-to-face working relationship between clients and case managers. Such a relationship is all-important, because case managers work with people who often feel the bite of stigma, discrimination, and isolation. It may be the only caring relationship some clients have available to them. For others, the case manager may offer the only hope of navigating a bureaucracy that might otherwise shuffle them around and neglect their needs. In any configuration, then, the case manager–client relationship must be given primary importance.[58]

Functional Elements and Role Definitions

Assessment, planning, intervention, monitoring, and evaluation are widely considered the core functions of case management[59] and are incorporated into professional standards guiding the execution of case management.[60,61] However, how these functions ultimately are implemented depends on the mission of the case management program; for example, in administratively driven programs the assessment function is provided by a gatekeeper, whereas client-driven programs depend on clients to assess their own needs and desires.

From a conceptual standpoint, a distinction can be made between direct and indirect intervention approaches.[62] In the *direct intervention approach,* the case manager works directly with clients to improve their skills in self-care, service acquisition, and self-monitoring. In some models, such as clinical case management or rehabilitation case management, direct intervention may take the form of counseling, psychotherapy, behavioral management, social skills training, or job search skills training.

The *indirect intervention approach* focuses the case manager's attention on systems intervention, including perhaps work with service systems, community gatekeepers, and families, with the aim of mustering needed service and social supports for clients.[63] Referral, linkage and brokering, advocacy, coordination, and consultation activities may be provided in conjunction with service systems, whereas social network interventions such as education, training, and support of significant others may be offered by the case management program. Implementation of the indirect intervention function may vary by programmatic mission. An administratively driven program may emphasize activities that enable it to control (through gatekeeping, monitoring, and evaluation) the delivery of services to clients. A program with a linkage and support mission may emphasize activities that result in the promotion and sustenance of social supports, self-help, and mutual assistance.

Actual programmatic experience with these assessment, planning, intervention, monitoring, and evaluation functions may diverge from idealized designs. For example, one comprehensive case management program is designed to fulfill all of these major functions. However, evaluative data reveal that the bulk of the program's effort is invested in crisis intervention — both directly with clients, in this case adolescents with serious emotional problems, and indirectly with family members, school officials, and community members. This divergence of intended case management functions from actual program experience underscores the need for ongoing evaluation of the characteristics and needs of the target population, levels of case management effort, actual functional activities and time commitments of case managers, and the achievement of specific program objectives.[64]

The selection and prioritization of case management functions will, like the program configuration, be influenced by the needs of the intended beneficiaries as well as by the mission of the program. For some functions, such as linkage to income maintenance or housing, case manager roles and assignments may be more strictly defined. This form of role specialization contrasts with a generalist approach in which all case managers undertake functions comprehensively with little specialization. The generalist approach may be more consistent with an individual configuration of case management than with a team configuration.

Service "Dosage"

The correct "dosage" of case management services, measured according to the frequency and duration of case management activities, can best be determined by the needs of the intended beneficiaries and the mission of the case management program.[65,66] Some situations require intensive case management, others require only minimal contact at set, fixed intervals.

In Assertive Community Treatment, for example, it is not unusual for case managers to interact with clients several times a week and to invest a considerable amount of time during each visit.[67] The mission here is to assist people with serious mental illness who are high utilizers of expensive services to live stable lives in the community. During periods of crisis or acute flare-ups of illness, case managers may be in daily contact with the client and significant others, especially if frequent monitoring is necessary.

On the other hand, in many mental health programs, case managers may see their clients only when their clients have appointments for medical reviews, medication updates, or milestone health visits. These case managers may schedule periodic client visits for these interventions.

Of course, the intensity of case management services may vary in any program. Activity may increase during periods of acuity and taper off during stable periods. Transitional points of service delivery, such as admission, transfer, or discharge, also may call for intensified case management activity.

Another critical dimension influencing case management dosage is an understanding of the specific impairment, illness, or disability that is the focus of the program. Every illness has its own trajectory of prodromal symptoms, acuity, stabilization, and decline. Sensitive case management programs will be designed to react flexibly to clients' changing needs.

Program Staffing

Actually staffing the case management program is a crucial step in the development of a program model. Will the case management program have a strong disciplinary identification? Will it have an interdisciplinary or transdisciplinary orientation? Or will it be deprofessionalized? The answers to these questions will have significant implications for program staffing.[68]

Staffing operationalizes the mission, purpose, and goals of the case management program. In outpatient programs, representatives of any qualified discipline—physicians, nurses, social workers, physical therapists, health educators, or counselors—can fulfill the role of case manager. If one discipline will dominate the staffing of the case management program, planners should consider what these individuals will be expected to achieve, their authority, and their power and respect within the health care organization.

For example, an outpatient service that cares for people with debilitating neurological problems may require nurses serving as case managers to have graduate degrees. But failing to address the perceived authority of these nurses among the program's physicians may cause conflicts between case managers and physicians. The medical staff may simply choose to bypass the case management function. Alternatively, the outpatient service may put in place a case management program to decrease unnecessary utilization linked to psychosocial conditions. Graduate-level social workers may be recruited to serve in case manager roles, but their integration into a medical setting may be attenuated by the friction between medical and social orientations to patient management.[69]

Interdisciplinary and transdisciplinary approaches may be introduced to reduce role conflict and competition among various health disciplines. In the *interdisciplinary approach,* program staffing may blend various professional disciplines, including medical consultation, nursing, social work, physical therapy, and rehabilitation counseling.[70] Given the proper programmatic framework, these disciplines can learn about one another's perspectives, cross-train, and collaborate to solve clients' problems. Some particularly effective interdisciplinary case management programs rotate case leadership; the professional who is most appropriate to a specific case takes primary case management responsibility. The *transdisciplinary approach* achieves this blend by original design, emphasizing recruitment of professionals with the most appropriate skills and experiences as opposed to specific credentials such as degrees. Both interdisciplinary and transdisciplinary approaches present challenges in terms of teamwork, team problem solving, systems thinking, conflict resolution, and communication and interpersonal support.[71]

With some success, researchers have explored the possibility of expanding the role of consumers, family members, and laypersons in case management activities.[72] Such deprofessionalization can be useful when case management tasks are routine, high levels of clinical judgment are not required, and these case managers are provided sound and timely supervision. As case managers, consumers offer a sensitivity to clients' problems and issues and a personal approach that professionals may not be able to offer. In addition, consumers may be more flexible in their execution of case management roles and more amenable to serving in community outreach roles, offering friendly visiting, providing support during periods of stress, assisting with transportation, and offering assistance in performing independent living activities.

For example, a program for elderly persons with complex health conditions may bring together an interdisciplinary case management team that combines both professional and nonprofessional staff—nurses, social workers, and rehabilitation specialists assisted by nondegreed case aides and volunteer family members. Such a program is able to offer its clients a full range of social support, linkage and access services, professional guidance and problem solving, and assistance with daily living needs.

Planners might wisely consider program staffing during the program configuration stage. It is important to remember that an effective case management program is built on a staff with the necessary knowledge, skills, and credentials to perform the functional activities its client population requires.[73]

• Additional Considerations

A program model is the fruition of the many steps and decisions that define the case management program's mission, configuration, functional elements and role definitions, service dosage, and staffing. There are no definitive rules for integrating all of these decisions into an effective model. Ongoing evaluation of the process and awareness of the ethical implications of the various phases of program development also are crucial to the program's success.

Ongoing Evaluation

Evaluation plays a vital role in every step of the case management program development process. Specifically, the initial stages of program development entail four levels of evaluation:

1. *Context evaluation:* This is an evaluation of consumer needs, stakeholder perspectives, and policy, administrative, and regulatory requirements as well as the various environments and settings in which the case management program will operate. Context evaluation is a predesign step.
2. *Input evaluation:* This is an evaluation of the necessary facilities, equipment, staffing, and organizational arrangements under consideration. Input evaluation comes into play when developers are actually designing the program.
3. *Process evaluation:* This is an evaluation of whether the program is functioning according to the original design and with the desired attributes. Process evaluation occurs during program implementation.
4. *Product evaluation:* This is an evaluation of the actual outcomes, effects, and impacts of the case management program.

All of these forms of evaluation will require program developers to revisit the program's mission, purpose, and goals.

Hidden Ethical Implications

Considering the rich diversity of program purposes, approaches, and arrangements in outpatient case management today, program development is largely a matter of choice. But before a choice can be made, program developers must first assess the specific needs of the program and its clients and then examine a number of options and synthesize a suitable program design. But program developers must beware! The simplest choices have the most serious ethical implications for outpatient health services seeking to develop relevant and meaningful case management programs.

Many of the ethical dilemmas in the case management field are tied to the innovative nature and sometimes misunderstood aims of these programs. To clarify matters, case managers should obtain potential clients' informed consent, fully explaining the strengths and limitations of case management service delivery and the true aims of the program. For example, when being asked to participate in an administratively driven case management program, clients should be apprised of the program's rationing and cost containment goals[74] and the possibility of "mixed loyalties." (With such a strong programmatic emphasis on cost control, will case managers be loyal to the consumer or to the organization for which they control costs?)

Outpatient health services must consider the program's potential conflicts of interest, a contingency about which all clients should be informed. Such disclosure empowers clients with as much information as possible so that they have the following:

1. A clear definition of case management procedures (such as making contacts with significant others to assess levels of social support)
2. Knowledge of the risks and benefits involved in case management (such as the possibility of rationing some forms of care or diverting consumers to new forms of service)
3. The possibility of conflicts of interest (such as being responsive to administrative mandates and not the desires of consumers)
4. An understanding of client rights within the case management system (such as opportunity to lodge a formal complaint against the case management service)

A linkage and support case management model is not exempt from ethical dilemmas. First, clients may need to understand the policies and procedures that guide disclosure of medical, psychological, behavioral, and social information to other agencies and that guarantee preservation of the client's privacy. Second, the program's emphasis on the organization of social supports on behalf of clients also needs to be disclosed; the client must understand the potential burdens, conflicts, and problems inherent in such procedures. Third, significant others also should be fully apprised, because social support procedures can create burdens they may not anticipate or can force them to assume responsibilities they may not wish to assume. Linkage and support models may shift the health care burden from provider to family members, sometimes as a conscious strategy by the sponsor of the case management program to shift or share costs. Even if cost shifting or cost sharing is unintentional, secondary consumers should be alerted to this contingency and be fully informed about the potentially stressful burden they are agreeing to assume as primary caregivers.

The dilemma of mixed loyalties also can emerge in the linkage and support model if case managers are paid directly by families to serve a dependent family member.[75] Under these circumstances, to whom is the case manager ultimately responsible—the family or the client?

The client-driven case management model's ethical implications lie in its emphasis on self-determination, empowerment, and autonomy. Given the choice, some individuals may not want to carry such responsibility on their own, preferring that professionals make critical decisions for them.[76] Of course, there are precedents for such relationships in attorney–client and physician–

patient advocacy. But case managers in client-driven models must strive to distinguish clients who have legitimately assigned their rights of autonomy and self-determination to others from those who merely lack motivation or commitment to participating in their own care. Declining to serve clients in the latter group may place clients in the former group at risk of serious neglect.

Pluralistic Approach to Program Development

There is no simple way to resolve these ethical dilemmas, but the outpatient health care service might well begin by implementing policies and procedures that clarify the program mission, clearly define case manager roles, and provide third-party protection of clients' rights.

A planning approach that involves many stakeholders also can assist the outpatient service in forming a program with strong legitimacy and the ability to navigate ethical challenges as they arise. The case management program can potentially link to its host organization, other human service systems and providers, family members, clients who may have serious disabilities, and community gatekeepers. Involving all these stakeholders in the program development process will ensure that the resulting model has the requisite inputs and a meaningful relevance to multiple consumers. Although the case management program's ultimate consumers will be its clients, many other groups may rightfully expect certain outcomes from the program.

• Conclusion

Program development involves many key decisions, a healthy amount of discourse, and perhaps inevitably, some turf battles. Setting meaningful goals and pursuing those goals in a logical, stepwise development process, case management program planners can sidestep the most common pitfalls.

A program design that embraces a principal foundation or perspective (such as the consumer's) may eliminate controversy during planning, but conflict will emerge early in the implementation process as different stakeholder groups attempt to shape the program to meet their own preferences and values. Involving multiple perspectives and disciplines early in program design is a strategy for successful, supportive program implementation.

Seizing the opportunity to excel in outpatient case management—the fastest-growing area of health delivery in contemporary practice—will require systematic planning, a committed development process, and frequent evaluation and modification. But the investment of time and effort will pay big dividends, not least among them the rewards of providing a broad spectrum of resources to serve clients with complex needs.

References

1. Freddolino, P., Moxley, D., and Fleishman, J. A field tested advocacy model for people with long term psychiatric disabilities. *Hospital and Community Psychiatry* 40(11):1169–74, 1989.

2. Dill, A. Issues in case management for the chronically mentally ill. In: D. Mechanic, editor. *Improving Mental Health Services: What the Social Sciences Can Tell Us.* San Francisco: Jossey-Bass, 1987, pp. 61–70.

3. Netting, F. E. Case management: service or symptom? *Social Work* 37(2):160–64, 1992.

4. Applebaum, R., and Austin, C. *Long-Term Case Management: Design and Evaluation.* New York City: Springer, 1990.

5. Arkansas Department of Human Services, Office on Aging. Comprehensive case management guidelines. Little Rock, AR: Arkansas Department of Human Services, 1984.

6. Bachrach, L. The chronic patient: Case management revisited. *Hospital and Community Psychiatry* 40(9):883–84, 1989.

7. Baerwald, A. Case management. In: L. Wikler and M. P. Keenan, editors. *Developmental Disabilities: No Longer a Private Tragedy.* Silver Spring, MD: National Association of Social Workers, 1983, pp. 219–23.

8. Baier, M. Case management with the chronically mentally ill. *Journal of Psychosocial Nursing and Mental Health Services* 25(6):17–20, 1987.

9. Brindis, C., Barth, R. P., and Loomis, A. B. Continuous counseling: case management with teenage parents. *Social Casework* 68:164–72, 1987.

10. Cheung, K., Stevenson, K., and Leung, P. Competency-based evaluation of case management skills in child sexual abuse intervention. *Child Welfare* 70(4):425–35, 1991.

11. Cohen, A., and Degraaf, B. Assessing case management in the child abuse field. *Journal of Social Service Research* 5(1,2):29–43, 1982.

12. Davis, I. Client identification and outreach: case management in school-based services for teenage parents. In: B. Vourlekis and R. Greene, editors. *Social Work Case Management.* New York City: Aldine, 1992.

13. Dixon, T., Goll, S., and Stanton, K. Case management issues and practices in head injury rehabilitation. *Rehabilitation Counseling Bulletin* 31(4):325–43, 1988.

14. Like, R. C. Primary care case management: a family physician perspective. *Quality Review Bulletin* 14(6):174–78, 1988.

15. Susser, M., Hopper, K., and Richman, J. Society, culture, and health. In: D. Mechanic, editor. *Handbook of Health, Health Care, and the Health Professions.* New York City: Free Press, 1983, pp. 23–49.

16. Institute of Medicine. *Disability in America.* Washington, DC: National Academy Press, 1991.

17. Moxley, D. *The Practice of Case Management.* Newbury Park, CA: Sage, 1989.

18. Harris, M., and Bachrach, L. *Clinical Case Management.* San Francisco: Jossey-Bass, 1988.

19. Roessler, R., and Rubin, S. *Case Management and Rehabilitation Counseling.* Baltimore: University Park Press, 1982.

20. Wray, L., and Wieck, C. Moving persons with developmental disabilities toward less restrictive environments through case management. In: K. Lakin and R. Bruininks, editors. *Strategies for Achieving Community Integration of Developmentally Disabled Citizens.* Baltimore: Paul H. Brookes, 1985.

21. Barker, R. L. *Case Management: Social Work Dictionary.* Silver Spring, MD: National Association of Social Workers, 1987.

22. Moxley, D., and Freddolino, P. Needs of homeless people coping with psychiatric problems: findings from an innovative advocacy project. *Health and Social Work* 16:19–26, 1991.

23. McKnight, J. Organizing the community. In: M. Linz, P. McAnally, and C. Wieck, editors. *Case Management: Historical, Current, and Future Perspectives.* Cambridge, MA: Brookline, 1989.

24. Freddolino, P., Moxley, D., and Fleishman, J. Daily living needs at time of discharge: implications for advocacy. *Psychosocial Rehabilitation Journal* 11(4):33–46, 1988.

25. Berk, R. A., and Rossi, P. H. *Thinking about Program Evaluation.* Newbury Park, CA: Sage, 1990.

26. Peterson, C. P. L. 99-457 — Challenges and changes for early intervention. In: M. Linz, P. McAnally, and C. Wieck, editors. *Case Management: Historical, Current, and Future Perspectives.* Cambridge, MA: Brookline, 1989.

27. National Association of Social Workers. *Case Management in Health, Education, and Human Services Settings.* Washington, DC: NASW, 1992.

28. Rose, S. *Case Management and Social Work Practice.* New York City: Longman, 1992.

29. Bachrach, L. Continuity of care for chronic mental patients: a conceptual analysis. *American Journal of Psychiatry* 138(11):1449–56, 1981.

30. Granet, R., and Talbot, J. The continuity agent: creating a new role to bridge the gaps in the mental health system. *Hospital and Community Psychiatry* 29:132–33, 1978.

31. Parker, M., and Secord, L. J. Case managers: guiding the elderly through the health care maze. *American Journal of Nursing* 88(12):1674–76, 1988.

32. Intagliata, J. Improving the quality of community care for the chronically mentally disabled: the role of case management. *Schizophrenia Bulletin* 8(4):655–74, 1982.

33. Baker, F., and Weiss, R. The nature of case manager support. *Hospital and Community Psychiatry* 35:925–28, 1984.

34. Skarnulis, E. Issues in case management for the '90s. In: M. Linz, P. McAnally, and C. Wieck, editors. *Case Management: Historical, Current, and Future Perspectives.* Cambridge, MA: Brookline, 1989.

35. Moxley, D., and Freddolino, P. A model of advocacy for promoting client self-determination in psychosocial rehabilitation. *Psychosocial Rehabilitation Journal* 14(2):69–82, 1990.

36. Ashley, A. Interdisciplinary update: case management — the need to define goals. *Hospital and Community Psychiatry* 39(5):499–500, 1988.

37. Witkin, B. R. *Assessing Needs in Educational and Social Programs.* San Francisco: Jossey-Bass, 1984.

38. Netting.

39. Baker, F., and Intagliata, J. Rural community support services for the chronically mentally ill. *Journal of Community Psychology* 5:3–14, 1984.

40. DeWeaver, K. L., and Johnson, P. L. Case management in rural areas for the developmentally disabled. *Human Services in the Rural Environment* 8(4):23–31, 1983.

41. Rothman, J. *Guidelines for Case Management: Putting Research to Professional Use.* Itasca, IL: Peacock, 1992.

42. Rothman.

43. Rapp, C. The strengths perspective of case management with persons suffering from severe mental illness. In: D. Saleebey, editor. *The Strengths Perspective in Social Work Practice.* New York City: Longman, 1992.

44. Moxley.

45. NASW.

46. Steinberg, R. M., and Carter, G. W. *Case Management and the Elderly.* Lexington, MA: Lexington, 1983.

47. Abrahams, R., and Leutz, W. The consolidated model of case management to the elderly. *Pride Institute Journal of Long-Term Health Care* 6(4):29–34, 1983.

48. Gottesman, L. E., Ishizaki, B., and MacBride, S. M. Service management: plan and concept in Pennsylvania. *The Gerontologist* 19(4):379–85, 1979.

49. Granet and Talbot.

50. Gerhard, R., Dorgan, R., and Miles, D. *The Balanced Service System.* Clinton, OK: Responsive Systems Associates, 1981.

51. Barker.

52. Levine, I., and Fleming, M. *Human Resource Development: Issues in Case Management.* Washington, DC: National Institute of Mental Health, 1984.

53. Ducanis, A. J., and Golin, A. K. *The Interdisciplinary Health Care Team.* Germantown, MD: Aspen, 1979.

54. Moxley.

55. Freddolino, Moxley, and Fleishman. Field tested advocacy model for people with long term psychiatric disabilities.

56. Rapp, C., and Wintersteen, R. The strengths model of case management: results from twelve demonstrations. *Psychosocial Rehabilitation Journal* 13(1):23–32, 1989.

57. Bond, G., Pensec, M., Dietzen, L., McCafferty, D., Giemza, R., and Sipple, H. Intensive case management for frequent users of psychiatric hospitals in a large city: a comparison of team and individual caseloads. *Psychosocial Rehabilitation Journal* 15(1):90–97, 1991.

58. Rapp.

59. Rubin, A. Case management. *Encyclopedia of Social Work* 18:212–22, 1987.

60. NASW.

61. Rose.

62. Moxley.

63. Moxley.

64. First, R. J., Greenlee, R. W., and Schmitz, C. A qualitative study of two community treatment teams. Summary Report. Columbus, OH: Ohio Department of Mental Health, 1990.

65. Bond, G., Miller, L., Krumwied, R., and Ward, R. Assertive case management in three CMHCs: a controlled study. *Hospital and Community Psychiatry* 39(4):411–18, 1988.

66. Rog, D., Andranovich, G., and Rosenblum, S. *Intensive Case Management for Persons Who Are Homeless and Mentally Ill: A Review of Community Support Program and Human Resource Development Program Efforts.* Washington, DC: Cosmos Corporation, 1987.

67. Eggert, G. M., Friedman, B., and Zimmer, J. Models of intensive case management. *Journal of Gerontological Social Work* 15(3,4):75–101, 1990.

68. Levine and Fleming.

69. Mizrahi, T., and Abramson, J. Sources of strain between physicians and social workers: implications for social workers in health care settings. *Social Work in Health Care* 10(3):33–51, 1985.

70. Wodarski, L. A., Bundschuh, E., and Forbus, W. Interdisciplinary case management: a model for intervention. *Journal of the American Dietetic Association* 88(3):332–35, 1988.

71. Senge, P. *The Fifth Discipline.* New York City: Doubleday, 1990.

72. Seltzer, M., Ivry, J., and Litchfield, L. Family members as case managers: partnership between the formal and informal support networks. *The Gerontologist* 27(6):722–28, 1987.

73. Moxley, D., and Buzas, L. Perceptions of case management services for elderly persons. *Health and Social Work* 14(3):196–203, 1989.

74. Kane, R. A. Case management: ethical pitfalls on the road to high quality managed care. *Quality Review Bulletin* 14(5):161–66, 1988.

75. Kane.

76. Rothman.

Chapter 5

The Emergence of Case Management Models

Elaine M. Sampson

• Introduction

The national agenda for health care reform promises to forge an integrated delivery system through bold legislation, a complete overhaul of reimbursement patterns, and profound changes in provider–consumer relations. Hospitals, insurers, physicians, vendors, professionals, paraprofessionals, and patients all will experience significant fallout as these major transformations are phased in over the next decade. Combined with rapidly advancing technologies, economic and quality incentives, and other payer initiatives, such sweeping changes command an innovative and swift response. Health care organizations will have to shorten their learning curves and become more responsive just to keep pace.

In the outpatient arena, keeping pace will require development of creatively designed and carefully implemented case management programs. Providing care in nontraditional ways — removed from inpatient settings, often using new technology — outpatient providers will have to find new ways to promote access, ensure quality, and control costs, and to help a diverse patient/family population navigate a complex and fragmented care continuum. The success of health care reform will depend on how well outpatient case management and other innovative delivery programs can answer these challenges in communities across the country.

This chapter describes the two emerging types of case management — fiscal and clinical — and how they relate to each other. It also offers five collaborative models of case management and emphasizes the role of nurses in the case management process as both case managers and program administrators. Finally, this chapter examines the case management program's need to market its services to both physicians and customers as it carves its niche in the home health arena.

• The Practice and Promise of Outpatient Case Management

Case management offers continuity of care within the continuum of inpatient and outpatient service provision, with a focus on the needs of patients and their families. It already has been, and promises to continue as a driving force in health care reform.

Focus on Family and Community

The family unit is the focal point of outpatient case management. By offering services in the patient's home or at nearby facilities, case management helps families remain intact when one member suffers an acute or extended illness. The case management program also helps patients, families, payers, and various providers or vendors surmount the barriers between inpatient sites and the home or other form of community-based care.

The definition, practice, and function of case management varies according to care-giving or case-managing disciplines, reimbursement sources, and delivery sites. Frequently, a client may be assigned more than one kind of case manager, for example, a hospital-based case manager or discharge planner and a payer-based case manager. Upon discharge to an outpatient service, the hospital-based case manager may pass the baton to the outpatient program's case manager, capitalizing on community resources rather than hospital resources. Still, although care settings and case managers may change, the program's focus never strays from the patient and family.

Emphasis on Continuity of Care

Continuity of care is the common goal of all case management programs and models. Although case manager responsibilities and assignments often may depend on the client's point of entry into the health care system, continuity of care must be preserved at all times. In managing the delivery of patient-centered care across various alternate delivery systems, and for both acute and chronic illnesses, case management aspires to provide:

> . . . the systematic assurance of uninterrupted, integrated medical and psychosocial care of the patient, in accord with the patient's wishes, from assessment of symptoms in the prediagnostic period, throughout the phase of active treatment, and for the duration of posttreatment monitoring and/or palliative care.[1]

Figure 5-1 illustrates the case management mechanisms for achieving continuity of care within the full continuum of inpatient and outpatient services.

Figure 5-1. Framework for Continuity of Care

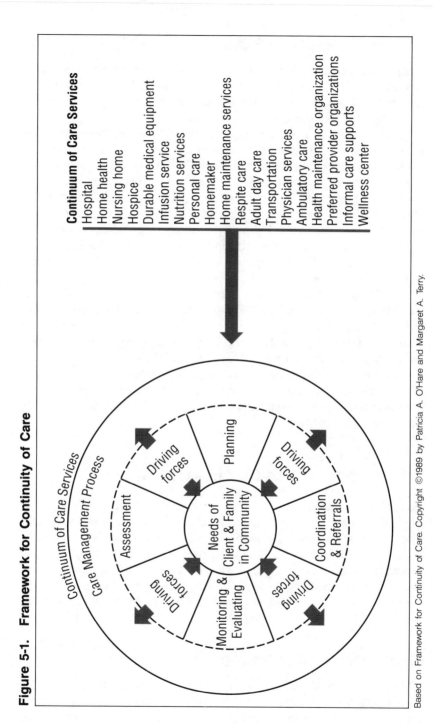

Continuum of Care Services

Care Management Process

Continuum of Care Services

Continuum of Care Services
Hospital
Home health
Nursing home
Hospice
Durable medical equipment
Infusion service
Nutrition services
Personal care
Homemaker
Home maintenance services
Respite care
Adult day care
Transportation
Physician services
Ambulatory care
Health maintenance organization
Preferred provider organizations
Informal care supports
Wellness center

Assessment

Planning

Driving forces

Driving forces

Driving forces

Driving forces

Needs of Client & Family in Community

Monitoring & Evaluating

Coordination & Referrals

Influence on Health Care Reform

Providers of outpatient case management services, especially home care agencies, are in a pivotal position to influence regional and national health care reform. The home care revolution has already effected important changes in federal health care policy.

Case management services now can be billed to Medicare under the guidelines covered in HIM-11, Management and Evaluation of the Care Plan, thanks to a lawsuit brought against the Health Care Financing Administration (HCFA) by a coalition of U.S. Congress members led by Representatives Harley Staggers (D-WV) and Claude Pepper (D-FL), consumer groups, and the National Association of Home Care (NAHC). The plaintiffs' victory in this lawsuit gave NAHC the opportunity to participate in rewriting Medicare's home health payment policies.[2] This has expanded the extent of services that can be considered reasonable and necessary for skilled care in the home care setting.

Skilled nursing visits for the management and evaluation of patient care plans are considered by HCFA to be reasonable and necessary when (1) underlying conditions or complications require a registered nurse to ensure that essential nonskilled care is achieving its purpose and (2) the complexity of the essential nonskilled care requires the involvement of skilled nursing personnel to promote recovery and medical safety in view of the patient's overall condition.[3] As home care and other case management initiatives take hold in our communities, they will wield even greater influence on the reform movement.

• Fiscal versus Clinical Case Management

As health care providers and payers have repositioned themselves to deliver high-quality, patient-centered acute care in shorter time frames, two distinct systems for case management have emerged: a fiscal (defensive) system and a clinical (offensive) system. The *fiscal case manager* is in the position of rationing the delivery of services, whereas the *clinical case manager* is in the position of justifying the need for services. These perspectives must be considered in concert to understand the tension that has grown between the two systems.

Fiscal (Defensive) Case Management

The primary goal of the fiscal case manager is to assist patients in securing their health coverage benefits in the most cost-effective, efficient manner. He or she determines what services the patient is eligible for and at what cost. In some cases, benefits will need to be expanded to cover the cost of a procedure or resource that was not included in the original contract, and the fiscal case manager must judge whether the additional coverage is justified.

The fiscal case manager also acts as a patient advocate. In this role, he or she reviews physician recommendations to ensure that reasonable and necessary treatment is being provided. In some cases, he or she may recommend that a second opinion be sought to prevent unnecessary treatment or surgery. This process regulates quality of care. In the execution of these responsibilities, the fiscal case manager also may discover health care professionals who have not acted in the best interest of the patient and report them to their professional organizations.

However, fiscal case managers may not have the education or expertise required to understand the implications of clinical treatment for complicated disease entities such as AIDS or cancer. Consequently, they are unable to fully consider patients' long-term needs or how future complications can be prevented by therapeutic measures today. Thus, nurses, for example, who do have the education and expertise to make such judgments, spend exorbitant amounts of time attempting to contact fiscal case managers for patient care updates and treatment authorizations.

Clinical (Offensive) Case Management

The primary goal of the clinical case manager is to identify the patient's physical and psychological needs and to secure the services that will enable the patient to achieve the desired outcome. The clinical case manager maneuvers the patient through the health care system and, practicing the fine art of negotiation, provides rationale as to why the services that have been requested are reasonable and necessary. At this point, the clinical case manager interacts with the fiscal case manager to determine what services the patient should receive.

Not every patient requires clinical case management. Normally, need is determined by the client's severity of illness, discharge status, service utilization (diagnosis-related group category), and availability of support systems. Clinical case managers must have a strong clinical background and highly specialized skills to coordinate and administer care and resources for oncology, AIDS, mental health, neonatology, and other focused patient populations with complex needs. Progressive hospitals have adopted product line approaches or critical care pathways to standardize clinical case management processes and to ensure high-quality care.

Health care professionals, who have spent so many years acquiring their valuable knowledge and experience, often are greatly frustrated by their lack of control and autonomy in rendering patient care and by endless, fruitless telephone conversations and paper chases. In the new paradigm for case management, health care professionals should be empowered to make decisions based on professional standards of care, critical pathways, or other care guidelines.

• The Strain of Case Management

The prospective payment strategies adopted by the federal government and private insurers have forever changed inpatient and outpatient care delivery systems. In the process, the shift toward outpatient care delivery has put considerable strain on all health care providers and has caused them to alter their practice patterns. The "quicker and sicker" discharge syndrome that evolved with diagnosis-related groups (DRGs) has snowballed into a managed care arrangement that is putting the squeeze on all hospital-based providers. The transition period has been very stressful and complicated by formidable barriers:

- Sick patients with complicated cases, but admitted for short hospital stays, are not allowed enough time to adjust to their illness, become knowledgeable about their care, and learn how to perform a new medical treatment or to take their prescribed medications.
- Inpatient health care providers, given less time to assess patients' psychological and social needs, may not be able to gather the information they need to prepare the family to participate in posthospital care.
- Families are not allowed the time they may need to rearrange their lives in order to care for family members. Employers, too, may not give employees time off to make arrangements for themselves or family members.
- Patients and families who perceive they are being hurried out of the health care system are angry and fearful about returning home.
- It is difficult to disseminate pertinent patient information to all the members of the health care team and to coordinate care-planning efforts in an alternate setting.
- Comprehensive data collected during the inpatient stay are not transmitted to outpatient providers on a timely basis.
- Hospital discharge planners burdened with heavy caseloads are constrained in their ability to complete a thorough assessment of patients' outpatient needs.
- Liability concerns have created a documentation nightmare. Health care professionals are required to submit reams of paperwork, which consumes far too much of their time.
- Home care agencies are being asked to accept patients and initiate service on shorter notice. In the rush, home health care professionals do not receive complete referral information from their inadequate information networks.

- Outpatient providers must obtain approval from payers before they can initiate service, hampering their ability to deliver care quickly in response to urgent patient needs.

• Five Collaborative Models of Case Management

The considerable strains placed on providers, payers, patients, and systems call for a strong collaborative relationship between inpatient caregivers, fiscal case managers, and clinical case managers. Case management programs can facilitate such collaboration through several models:[4]

1. *Broker model:* In this model, public or private not-for-profit organizations provide case management services to functionally impaired persons at risk of entering a nursing home; however, they have no (or limited) authority to purchase services for the clients. The case management agency serves a coordinating function and also may be a service provider. Usually, the full panoply of case management service is offered.
2. *Purchase authority model:* In this model, public or private not-for-profit organizations provide case management services to functionally impaired individuals who are eligible to receive community-based long-term care under Medicaid, Medicaid waivers, or some other publicly funded program, such as a state program, an Older American's Act program, or one using pooled funds.
3. *Capitated model:* Here, case management is provided within a health service model that is capitated for acute, ambulatory, and all long-term care services for voluntarily enrolled functionally able and disabled Medicare-eligible clients.
4. *Insurance model:* In conjunction with long-term care insurance, case management services are either contracted out or performed internally by the company to contain the total cost of the long-term care benefits provided under the plan.
5. *Fee-for-service model:* This model includes independent fee-for-service firms, either for-profit or not-for-profit, that vend case management services for private geriatric or nongeriatric clients. The firms are paid by their clients out-of-pocket.

With today's variety of ownership, organizational, and operational structures, a single case management program may employ several models. For example, a Medicare-certified home care agency with a for-profit arm provides case management services under at least three models: broker, purchase authority, and fee-for-service. In fact, any program may embrace any combination of the five models above, whether as a provider of acute or long-term care.[5] Table 5-1 compares the broker, purchase authority, capitated, insurance, and fee-for-service models in terms of their service features, program goals, reimbursement mechanisms, and constraints.

Table 5-1. Models of Case Management

Dimensions	Broker	Purchase Authority	Capitated	Insurance	Fee for Service
Service features					
Extent of integration:					
Case management only	X			X	X
Case management and community-based long-term care		X			
Case management community-based long-term care, and institutional care			X		
Case management functions					
Assessment, care planning, and monitoring	X				X[1]
Full spectrum case management		X			
Full spectrum case management and utilization review			X	X	
Goals[2]					
Minimize nursing home use	X				
Minimize nursing home use and efficient community-based long-term care use		X			
Minimize cost of case management, community-based long-term care, and institutional care			X	X	
Maximize profits and revenues					X
Reimbursement mechanisms					
Fixed budget	X	X			
Annual capitation			X	X[3]	
Administrative cost					
Fee-for-service and billable hours					X
Constraints					
Process that relates case management time to cost of community-based long-term care	X	X	X	X	
Process that relates community based long-term care use to institutional care use	X	X	X	X	
Fixed budget for case management	X	X			
Per client cap on community-based long-term care costs		X			
Private demand for case management					X

1 Private case manager may not do monitoring if client does not want to pay for that service feature.

2 All goals are qualified by implicit standards of care.

3 If case management is contracted out by insurance company, it may be a fee-for-service or capitated arrangement.

Source: R. A. Kane, J. D. Penrod, G. B. Davidson, I. Moscovice, and E. Rich. *Case Management Costs: Conceptual Models and Program Descriptions.* Prepared for Health Care Financing Administration, Minneapolis. University of Minnesota Health Policy Center, June 1989.

• The Role of Nurses in Case Management

Nurses are key players in the process of case management. In addition to being the obvious choice for clinical case management, clinical nurse specialists are educated and prepared to fill the role of case management program administrator.

The Nurse as Case Manager

Case management programs led by primary care nurses hold the most promise for managing continuity of care throughout various health care institutions and home care or community settings. Nursing professionals are quick to embrace a collaborative, interdisciplinary approach that balances both cost and quality. Case management is nothing new to the many community and public health nurses who have long coordinated care for diverse patient populations. Nurses have been case managers since the turn of the century.

Of course, the valuable contributions of social workers to the case management process cannot be underestimated. But more and more case management programs are recognizing that a broader-based expertise is required to understand and meet the multifaceted demands of today's outpatient population.[6] Although the social worker is an integral member of the health care team, case management functions — especially comprehensive medical and psychosocial evaluations — are best conducted by a licensed registered nurse.

Nurses are the ideal and appropriate choice for clinical case management because they have the medical background and clinical and organizational skills that are essential to managing patient care. Nurses as case managers also have a significant role to play in supporting and influencing physicians in altering their practice patterns to contain costs and improve quality. Just as the case management program is instrumental in coordinating services, it also should support the collaborative practice of all the members of the health care team.

In 1975, the American Nurses Association (ANA) published its position on the nurse's role in discharge planning from the acute care setting, stating that responsibility for continuity of care planning cannot be delegated. Further, the ANA acknowledged that social workers definitely have a role to play in assisting clients, initiating the referral process, and providing technical information about nursing care and procedures that will be needed after discharge.[7] The ANA's definition emphasizes clinical nursing judgment in a case management process that includes assessment, planning, implementation, and evaluation on an interactive level among nurses, other providers, clients, and their families. The ANA also identified a number of specific case management functions that rely on clinical nursing judgments, including case screening, client assessment, data analysis, coordination of community services and resources, and client education. The goals of this nurse-directed case management process are quality of care, reduced fragmentation of services, enhancement of the client's quality of life, and containment of costs.[8]

The Clinical Nurse Specialist

The substantial growth in hospital-based home care programs has paralleled the migration to the outpatient setting. According to HCFA, the total number of home care agencies doubled between 1979 and 1990. During this period, the number of hospital-based home care agencies increased by 350 percent. This explosive growth underscores the need to provide continuity of care between the inpatient setting and the community.

To take advantage of this growth opportunity, the hospital-based case management program needs to offer a full range of services that are well integrated within the hospital and the surrounding community. The added value of a case management program that can target specific patient populations and disease categories such as gerontology, oncology, AIDS, and mental health is attractive to hospitals as well as communities. The ability to design and implement credible programs that address the special, focused needs of these populations may be enhanced by placing a clinical nurse specialist in the role of administrator.

The master's-prepared clinical nurse specialist (CNS) has the advanced clinical and fiscal expertise to manage both cost and quality of care. Further, as an educator, clinical expert, researcher, and consultant, the CNS can administer the program and associated staff. In this light, the CNS becomes the consultant supervising a professional staff responsible for care delivery. Schull, Tosch, and Wood conducted a study in Dallas that described the impact of the CNS role on cost and quality outcomes among three patient populations.[9] Average length of stay (ALOS) and readmission rates were calculated for case-managed and non–case-managed clients in each patient population. The rather significant results of the study indicated a reduction in LOS, readmission rates, and emergency department visits among cases managed by CNSs.

As clinician and program manager, the CNS gives the home care agency or hospital-based case management program a competitive advantage. Organizationally, he or she acts as liaison between the hospital and the home care agency or outpatient resource so that continuity of care is preserved. The CNS can be instrumental in assisting inpatient caregivers and hospital administrators in managing specific DRG categories that may be problematic in terms of LOS, rate of readmission, and utilization of services. In some settings, the clinical nurse specialist may act as product line manager for a specific patient population in collaboration with the administrator or unit leader for the agency.

The CNS administrator needs to develop a close working relationship with inpatient caregivers and physicians. Communication of pertinent information to the health care team is the key to continuity of care, and as administrator and liaison, the CNS plays a vital role in coordinating resources and providers to enhance that care.

• Tools for Marketing Case Management

In many instances, case managers are in the position of having to market the case management process to both physicians and outpatient clients. Many tools can be used to carry out this activity. These include opening communication, developing feedback mechanisms, tearing down barriers to outpatient access, and eliciting physician participation.

Facilitating Communication

Effective written and verbal communication is a powerful marketing tool. Every time a staff member writes, calls, or visits a customer, he or she makes a lasting impression. The clinical nurse specialist (CNS) sets the stage by facilitating the communication process. By attending discharge rounds and clinical case conferences and conducting predischarge visits, the CNS can take a proactive approach to planning posthospital care. One expert suggests:

> It appears that a mechanism is needed for effectively communicating inpatient providers' suggestions to outpatient providers; interventions that demonstrated the most promise for decreasing readmission were those in which outpatient providers attended to patient needs identified by inpatient providers at discharge.[10]

The mechanism referred to above is a *discharge plan*. The CNS may be consulted by a discharge planner, a physician, or a nurse to establish a discharge plan that will decrease the inpatient LOS. Community nurses depend on receiving accurate referral information in a timely manner to lessen the chance of exacerbation of illness or readmission, and linking the patient to community resources such as transportation, homemaker services, or Meals-on-Wheels will enable the patient to go home earlier.

> Evidence suggests that the cost-effectiveness of interventions may be enhanced by targeting these to patients with high risk of readmission. This would allow providers to increase the intensity of strategies to reduce readmission, since a smaller reduction in readmission rates would be required to demonstrate cost-effectiveness. Thus, programs for elderly inpatients, a group known to consume high levels of resources through readmission, are especially needed.[11]

Establishing Feedback Mechanisms

Another step in facilitating communication is to set up feedback mechanisms once the patient is admitted to outpatient case management so that information about his or her progress can then be transmitted back to the inpatient caregivers and the physician. This not only enhances the quality of care being provided, but also strengthens the program's alliance with the hospital and the physician by building confidence. These small efforts also will make a big difference in the mind of the customer and will go a long way toward ensuring repeat business. Because time is so crucial to physicians, customizing the information they need according to their preferences will give the program an edge in the marketplace. It is important to acknowledge that, because they may have admitting privileges at several hospitals that use different agencies, physicians may not know which agency is caring for each patient. Upon admission, the case manager can simply fax the physician some preliminary information about the patient, such as diagnoses, medications, lab work, vital signs, and a brief assessment, which will give the physician the opportunity to validate the information and keep it for the medical record in his or her office.

One of the most important ways the CNS administrator can positively influence treatment and care outcomes is to establish a program that not only cares for the patient, but that also reports on the patient's progress to the physician and inpatient caregivers.

Tearing Down the Barriers to Outpatient Access

If barriers to discharge are encountered, the CNS consults with the physician, inpatient nurses, the family, the fiscal case manager, and community groups to resolve them. If safety or inadequate resources pose a problem, the patient is not discharged until alternative arrangements can be made. For example, in some cases, patients may not give the inpatient caregivers accurate information about their home environment or their support system. Once the patient is home, the community nurse may find an undesirable situation that warrants taking appropriate action. Barriers to access could include an unsafe home environment, inadequate support systems, a caregiver who is unable or unwilling to participate in the care, scarce community resources, or poor transportation. Social service arrangements linking the patient to appropriate community resources usually are made prior to discharge.

The literature suggests that 80 percent of all home care is provided by families.[12] Because the stress on the family, and especially on caregivers, can be devastating, community resources should be developed with state or local funding to provide programs such as respite care.

Eliciting Physician Participation

Reimbursement for case management under the resource-based relative value scale (RBRVS) is not attractive to most physicians, who prefer not to spend their time talking with patients for the sole purpose of coordinating and managing complex out-of-hospital care. Traditionally, those activities are addressed by other members of the health care team. This is a difficult adjustment for physicians, who are well versed in the diagnostic process but lost when it comes to identifying systems and resources that will support their practice. Once the patient is in the outpatient setting, beyond the purview of the hospital's interdisciplinary team, the physician may not recognize the patient's need for case-managed services.

Physician involvement in case management is influenced by both reimbursement issues and training. Educating physicians regarding the valuable extension of their practice through case-managed alternatives is a major marketing activity. Physicians desire information about how they can alter their practice patterns and respond to the changes in health care policy. They are particularly interested in home care and many, given financial incentives for their time, will participate. On occasion, physicians are willing to make a home visit because it is good medical practice; but the current unreasonable reimbursement rates for home care do little to encourage physician home visits.

To stimulate physician involvement in home care, the National Association for Home Care (NAHC) has adopted the position that the services a physician performs in managing the care of a home health patient should be billed and paid separately when the patient's treatment needs impose a substantial burden on the physician.[13] Case management is an interdisciplinary process that requires physician involvement first and foremost. The home care agency or hospital-based program needs to develop mechanisms that encourage partnerships with physicians. Practice guidelines, critical pathways, and care plans for ambulatory care are forthcoming and may assist case managers in their collaborative practice with physicians as well as in the administration of home care programs.

In addition, managers can educate staff and develop systems that streamline or automate both written documentation and verbal communication with physicians. For example, on-line computer systems to facilitate required signatures and verify case plans should lighten paperwork requirements, which currently are a burden to many physicians. High-quality service to physician offices is a major determinant of high-quality care to the patient and a precursor to enhanced relationships with physicians. The case management forum offers the structure for supporting physicians in their modification of practice patterns, as they seek to reduce cost and maintain quality of care in a redesigned health care delivery system. For example, as a result of having to spend less time on the telephone with the patient and family and less time coordinating care, the physician will have more time to dedicate to direct patient care.

In the mind of the consumer, home health care is an extension of the physician practice. Patient satisfaction and the supportive practice complements offered by high-quality home care services are a strong advantage that may enhance the physician relationship with the patient, the family, and the home care provider.

• The Demand for Case Management

The demand for case management is strong among both inpatient and outpatient providers, and home care agencies are in a dynamic position to capture a significant portion of the market share through hospital and community affiliations. Case management product lines can be offered to an extensive array of customers. Table 5-2 provides an overview of the home care agency's potential customers, their needs for and expectations of case management, and the products the agency might wisely offer to meet those needs and expectations.

The fee-for-service agencies that offer case management services for geriatric patients pose the greatest threat to community home care agencies due to their ability to provide added-value services such as live-in companions. The services in highest demand are homemaker and companion services that provide assistance with daily living, including transportation. If these services are not offered by the community through church or service organizations, the home care agency should develop them in order to maintain and improve its market share.

Marketing case management to special populations, such as the elderly and their children, through professional organizations, community agencies, and health providers in the community will provide premier visibility. Marketing plans that highlight the specific benefits or services of home care or case management for special patient groups, such as AIDS, oncology, ventilator-assisted, and postpartum patients, are particularly effective. Select affiliations and contracts with hospitals, retirement centers, employers, and physician group practices for case management services offer a strong advantage in the home care marketplace.

• Conclusion

An effective case management program is fast becoming a necessary component of outpatient care. And the demand for outpatient case management will only rise with the continued growth and expansion of the outpatient arena and the aging of the population. In the years ahead, the

Table 5-2.   Marketing the Case Management Program

Potential Customer	Needs/Expectations	Case Management Product
Managed care for an HMO that integrates both acute and long-term care in a capitated, prepayment system for Medicare beneficiaries	Reduce risk of nursing home placement for the frail elderly. Decrease hospitalization and utilization of services. Promote independence at home.	Provide long-term care through the case management Medicare benefit, with supplemental services authorized by the HMO that will prevent exacerbation of illness and utilization of inpatient services.
Hospitals	Decrease LOS/decrease financial penalties from third-party payers. Generate new sources of income in the outpatient arena. Stabilize patient referral base. Capture patient/family as a lifetime customer. Diversify services by providing a community outreach program. Improve image in the community. Encourage use of inpatient services that can be used in the outpatient area (e.g., laboratory service, pharmacy). Emphasize medical staff development and satisfaction. Package inpatient and outpatient services to create product lines that can then be offered to third-party payers.	Provide a comprehensive range of programs that can be vertically integrated within the inpatient setting to decrease LOS. Consultation by a clinical nurse specialist who can provide assistance in managing populations at risk for overutilization of inpatient services. Hospital-based home care agencies will facilitate continuity of care and keep the patient within the system. Provide the hospital with the ability to extend services into the community. Influence physician practice patterns through the agency's marketing efforts. Prevent unnecessary hospital readmissions.
Employers	Reduce employee absenteeism. Reduce the risk of disability.	Evaluate health risks pertaining to an employer's workforce and provide consultation in developing programs designed to reduce risks. Provide home care for family members so the employee can continue working.
Ambulatory Surgery Centers	Preadmission screening, evaluation, and preoperative teaching. Postoperative follow-up.	Design protocols for specific procedures to include those services that can be provided in the home. These services can be offered to ambulatory care centers for a set fee.
Retirement Centers	Prevent nursing home placement. Health care delivery on site would be a way of attracting residents. Availability of physicians to make house calls.	Offer a wellness program for the elderly. To prevent the exacerbation of illness, promote compliance and admission to an inpatient setting. Individual case management for residents who are at risk for nursing home placement. Facilitate physician home visits.
Physician Group Practices	Shift to outpatient arena. Diversify services to capture a larger patient population. Provide comprehensive, multidisciplinary care without incurring additional overhead expenses. Manage chronic illness in the community. Enhance patient satisfaction.	Provide a full range of services to the physician practices in the community setting. Facilitate physician productivity by decreasing the amount of time spent managing chronic illness with the benefits of case management.

challenge to maintain an easily accessible and navigable continuum of care will require even closer collaboration among the practices and disciplines involved in case management.

Seamless care delivery through case management is best achieved by establishing open lines of communication between professionals whose common goal is to provide patient-focused, cost-effective care. Any barriers to interdisciplinary practice, high-quality care, and program administration must be surmounted with practical strategies to promote collaboration, streamline systems, encourage productivity, and create new standards of care. Sophisticated information systems for data management and networking will offer interagency documentation, information relay, automated medical records, utilization review, and other functions to support case management efforts. But people must communicate and cooperate to make those systems work.

All the while, public policymakers will be escalating efforts to redesign the nation's health care delivery system. A hospital's success in these changing times will depend on its ability to apply innovative, interdisciplinary methods of care and resource management that focus on the family and the community. It is not enough to stand ready to act; the pace of reform will be too brisk even for the organization that can turn on a dime. Hospitals must shape their own futures by establishing sound outpatient case management programs today.

References

1. Lauria, M. Continuity of cancer care. *Cancer* 67(suppl. 6):1759–66, 1991.

2. National Association of Home Care Agencies.

3. Health Care Financing Administration. *Health Care Insurance Manual-11.* (HIM-11). Rev. 222. Washington, DC: HFCA, 1989.

4. Davidson, G. B., Penrod, J. D., Kane, R. A., Moscovice, I. S., and Rich, E. C. Modeling the costs of case management in long term care. *Health Care Financing Review* 13(1):75–78, 1991.

5. Davidson and others.

6. McIntosh, L. Hospital-based case management. *Nursing Economics* 5(5):232–36, 1987.

7. Cooke, P. S., and Alley, J. M. Discharge planning: whose responsibility is it? *Caring,* Jan. 1992, pp. 28–32.

8. American Nurses Association. *Task Force on Case Management in Nursing: Nursing Care Management.* Kansas City, MO: ANA, 1988.

9. Schull, D. E., Tosch, P., and Wood, M. Clinical nurse specialists as collaborative care managers. *Nursing Management* 23(3):30–33, 1992.

10. Weinberg, M., and Oddone, E. Strategies to reduce hospital readmissions: a review. *Quarterly Review Bulletin* 15(8):255–59, 1989.

11. Weinberg and Oddone.

12. Gurland, B., Dean, L., Gurland, R., and Cook, D. The dependent elderly in New York City. *Community Council of Greater New York,* 1988.

13. Boling, A., and Keenan, J. M. Policy issues for physicians involved in home care. *Caring,* May 1992, pp. 4–12.

Bibliography

American Hospital Association. *Ambulatory Care Trendlines: Growth Trends in Hospital Home Care 1980–1990.* Eric Linnie, editor. Vol. 1, No. 3. Chicago: AHA, July 1992, p. 1–11.

American Nurses Association. *Task Force on Case Management in Nursing: Nursing Case Management.* Kansas City, MO: ANA, 1988.

Boling, P. A., and Keenan, J. M. Policy issues for physicians involved in home care. *Caring,* May 1992, pp. 4–12.

Christianson, J. B., Applebaum, R., Carcagon, G., and Phillips, B. Organizing and delivering case management services: lessons from the National Long Term Care Channeling Demonstration. *Home Health Care Services Quarterly* 9(1):7–27, 1988.

Cook, P. S., and Alley, J. M. Discharge planning: whose responsibility is it? *Caring,* Jan. 1992, pp. 28–32.

Davidson, G. B., Penrod, J. D., Kane, R. A., Moscovice, I. S., and Rich, E. C. Modeling the costs of case management in long-term care. *Health Care Financing Review* 13(1):73–81, Fall 1991.

Halamandaris, V. J. The paradox of case management. *Caring,* Aug. 1990, pp. 4–55.

Hereford, R. W. Private-pay case management: let the seller beware. *Caring,* Aug. 1990, pp. 8–12, Aug. 1990.

Jowett, S., and Armitage, S. Hospital and community liaison links in nursing: the role of the liaison nurse. *Journal of Advanced Nursing* 13(suppl. 6):579–87, 1988.

Lauria, M. M. Continuity of cancer care. *Cancer* 67:1759–66, 1991.

McIntosh, L. Hospital-based case management. *Nursing Economics* 5(5):232–36, 1987.

O'Hare, P. A., and Terry, M. A. Community-based care management: a framework for delivery of services. *Home Healthcare Nurse* 9(3):26–32, 1989.

Olivas, G. S., Tongno-Armanasco, V. D., Erickson, J. R., and Harter, S. Case management: a bottom-line care delivery model part 1: the concept. *Journal of Nursing Administration* 19(11):16–20, 1989.

Phillips, B. R., Kemper, P., and Applebaum, R. A. The evaluation of the National Long Term Care Demonstration. *Health Service Research* 23(1):67–81, 1988.

Pierog, L. J. Case management: a product line. *Nursing Administration Quarterly* 15(2):16–21, 1991.

Schroer, K. Case management: clinical nurse specialist and nurse practitioner, converging roles. *Clinical Nurse Specialist* 5(4):189–94, 1991.

Schull, D. E., Tosch, P., and Wood, M. Clinical nurse specialists as collaborative care managers. *Nursing Management* 23(3):30–32, 1992.

Shuster, G. F. III, and Cloonan, P. Nursing activities and reimbursement in clinical management. *Home Healthcare Nurse* 7(5):10–15, 1988.

Weinberg, M., and Oddone, E. Strategies to reduce hospital readmissions: a review. *Quarterly Review Bulletin* 15(8):255–59, 1989.

Weinstein, R. Hospital case management: the path to empowering nurses. *Pediatric Nursing* 17(3):289–93, 1991.

Chapter 6

Case Management and the Continuum of Care

Gerry Brueckner and Talar Glover

• Introduction

Providing high-quality, cost-effective health care today means harnessing the unruly variety of services and resources available in acute, skilled, and ambulatory care settings. As these services and resources have stretched beyond hospital walls and into our communities, so has the need to coordinate patient care. Health care organizations need a way to reclaim control over scattered patient populations that, for some, have become unmanageable.

Indeed, the success of health care reform may hinge on our ability to establish a process of comprehensive patient care that is both accessible and navigable from any point of entry. This ideal is commonly called the *continuum of care,* a term used so loosely these days that it is all but meaningless. So it is important to begin by establishing a stricter working definition:

> A *continuum of care* is an integrated system or package of health care support services that assures comprehensive, coordinated care for patients based on individualized service needs. At the same time, it guides and tracks patients over time through a comprehensive array of physical health, mental health, and social services spanning all levels of intensity, and includes both services and integrating mechanisms.

Chief among the continuum's "integrating mechanisms" is case management. Well-designed and consistently dependable case management programs will be the key to achieving a true continuum of care as reforms are phased in and as patients and services continue their migration to the outpatient arena.

This chapter describes how case management provides a communication link between the inpatient and outpatient providers involved in any individual patient's continuum of care. It also provides examples of successful service line integration and discusses how comprehensive care plans work.

• The Evolution of the Care Continuum

In recent years, a number of factors have had a hand in creating the current shift from inpatient to outpatient care, resulting in an expansion of the continuum of care to serve a new patient population. The following subsections describe how the shift evolved and how outpatient services are being incorporated into the patient's overall continuum of care.

Serving a Changing Patient Population

Considering how the efforts of so many, in so many different disciplines and facilities, must be orchestrated to serve patients' many individual needs, it is no wonder the U.S. health care delivery system has grown complex and fragmented. Just 10 years ago, before Medicare established its prospective payment system, things were simpler. The delivery system extended from the physician's office or the emergency department to the acute care hospital. With few exceptions, the delivery system included only two other settings: patients' homes, which social workers and public health nurses might visit to provide assessment, intervention, evaluation, or referrals; and nursing homes, some of which also provided short-term rehabilitation services.

Over the past decade, the continuum naturally has followed the shift from inpatient to outpatient care. As Medicare's fixed reimbursement scheme, in concert with numerous other payer initiatives and advancing technology, forced acute care facilities to work faster clinically if they wanted to maintain the bottom line financially, innovative care alternatives soon had to be developed to serve a new patient population.

To facilitate the earlier but safe discharge of patients from the hospital to more appropriate settings, the industry scrambled to create new roles such as discharge planners, care coordinators, and case managers. Hospital medical staffs formed multidisciplinary utilization review teams to monitor lengths of stay, the course and appropriateness of treatment, and discharge procedures. The Health Care Financing Administration established professional review organizations (PROs) to monitor inpatient management by physicians and hospital staff. And last, but not least, payers mandated admission criteria for specific services, supplying their own case managers and making their own recommendations for achieving a continuum of care. Some even began requiring preauthorization for elective procedures and rationed other services. Health maintenance organizations (HMOs) controlled access to the care continuum through physician "gatekeepers." In short, a new reality of health care delivery evolved.

In the aftermath of these industrywide shifts, obtaining truly comprehensive health care with any continuity poses a significant challenge for patients, their families, hospitals, physicians, and payers alike.

Braiding Outpatient Services into the Continuum

The levels of service available in the outpatient arena mirror their inpatient counterparts, as shown in figure 6-1. Actual treatment regimens may vary among inpatient and outpatient providers, and certain services for episodic illness, injury, and maintenance are provided in the outpatient setting only. Figure 6-2 lists a number of outpatient services and resources and places them on the continuum according to level of service.

A true continuum of care can only be accomplished by making available the entire spectrum of delivery sites, ranging from acute care and skilled nursing facilities to day hospitals, hospital-based therapy units, short-stay or recovery centers, and hospice and home care. Likewise, health care organizations need to tear down all barriers—operational, organizational, communicational, and financial—that divide patient care in hospitals from patient care in alternative settings. This concept of a "hospital without walls" is no longer considered revolutionary, but evolutionary.

Even though more effective, less costly outpatient interventions may be available, old ways of thinking often still guide the patient into an unnecessary and costly hospital stay. Because the criteria for outpatient care unfortunately have not yet been as clearly defined as have the criteria for inpatient admission, outpatient services are not always selected for all the right reasons; rather, they occur simply by default—that is, clients who do not meet inpatient admission criteria are referred to outpatient services. Most hospitals currently use Medicare PRO (diagnosis-specific) admission, treatment, and/or discharge criteria.

Ideally, a patient's course of treatment would be determined solely according to the efficacy and appropriateness of care to meet his or her needs. By defining the appropriate level of care and assigning the resources or services that best meet the client's needs, the admissions process should pinpoint the client's entry into a health care continuum that weighs inpatient and outpatient services equally. Whatever his or her point of entry, the client's further progress through the continuum must also be determined solely by specific clinical and personal needs, and the continuum of services must be comprehensive and flexible enough to accommodate a course of treatment that changes as client needs change. Clients should be eased toward the self-care end of the continuum as their conditions improve and, conversely, referred back toward total care should they suffer any serious setbacks or complications.

• Communication: The Key to Coordinating Services

With more and more consumers and payers selecting ambulatory care alternatives, coordination of these services has become a challenge. Escalating

Figure 6-1.   Continuum of Health Care Services

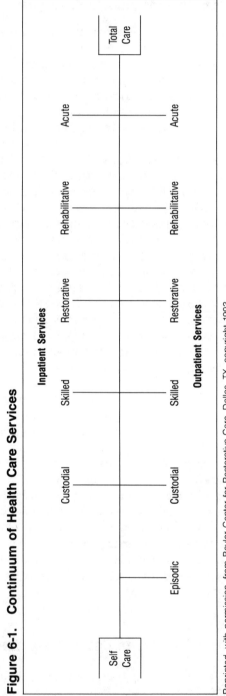

Reprinted, with permission, from Baylor Center for Restorative Care, Dallas, TX, copyright 1993.

Figure 6-2. Continuum of Outpatient Services and Resources

Level on Continuum	Outpatient Service/Resource
Acute	Outpatient surgery center Emergency department Minor emergency center Home care
Rehabilitative	Outpatient therapy Home therapy
Restorative	Home therapy Outpatient therapy
Skilled	Home care Hospice Infusion/Dialysis center
Custodial	Homemaker services Home-delivered meals Day care Primary/family care services
Episodic	Physician office Outpatient clinic

costs, stifling regulations, dwindling facility staffs, and eroding financial resources prompted the flight from the hospital; but without careful planning, ambulatory care settings may soon suffer the same plagues. As usual, the key is communication.

By shortening the total length of stay or circumventing the need for a hospital stay altogether, outpatient care services became an attractive alternative to traditional hospital care under a tighter reimbursement scheme. In bucking the tradition, though, caregivers and program managers cannot discard the tried and true lines of communication so essential to sound patient care planning. When hospital inpatients are discharged to outpatient settings or when ambulatory patients are shuffled between delivery sites, a brand-new kind of interdisciplinary communication is essential. Providers who share patients must share patient information, too. Lack of communication between professionals and between systems can result in:

• Prolonged morbidity
• Inappropriate resource utilization
• Duplication or fragmentation of services
• Increased cost

And more tragic scenarios certainly can be imagined, all of them avoidable with proper communication.

Case management provides a vital communication link between the many inpatient and outpatient providers in today's expanding continuum of care. The case management program can ensure that all caregivers have ready access to the complete, up-to-date patient information they need to play their important roles in the client's progress. Carefully documented medical records, usually kept handy at the patient bedside in the hospital setting, should be entrusted to the hands of mobile caregivers or reside with the hospital- or agency-based case manager. Any changes in the client's condition should promptly be telephoned in to the case manager. Any changes in case manager assignments should be relayed immediately to all providers on the case.

Always with a focus on the client's needs, the case manager recommends service referrals based on three factors:

1. *Physical:* How many and what types of services does the client need? Might the client's physical condition limit the choice of an appropriate care site? Is the client particularly frail or homebound?
2. *Psychosocial:* Is transportation a problem? Is a solid family support system in place?
3. *Financial:* What is the client's ability to pay? Who will be the payer(s)?

Ensuring that caregivers in the field fully communicate this physical, psychosocial, and financial information to the responsible case manager is the surest way to chart a prudent, effective, and economical course of treatment in a variety of settings.

Large health care systems enjoy the natural advantage of being able to provide the entire service spectrum in a unified continuum of care. The centralized administration and usually close proximity of system-based sites provide an excellent environment for communication and coordinated care. In addition, systems can realize greater economies of scale in purchasing and staffing and can provide a greater variety and complexity of services.

Nonsystem institutions are trying to catch up, but for some, vertical organizational and accountability structures have laid parallel tracks that never cross. Disciplines that must cooperate in daily clinical practice may work together side by side but with little or no communication in the planning and provision of patient care. When departments and caregivers are put at cross purposes, the resulting fragmentation of the organizational infrastructure prohibits the advancement of a continuum.

• The Integration of Service Lines

In creating ambulatory care systems, poorly structured organizations replicate their poor organizational structures. Historically, the average health care organization discourages the horizontal integration of departments, such as home care and ambulatory surgery, that operate under different administrators. Integrating these service lines — inpatient to inpatient, inpatient to outpatient, and outpatient to outpatient — is a matter of sharing vital patient care information and responsibilities.

Today, with dramatically shorter inpatient stays, hospitals are ready, even eager, to "marry" their inpatient and outpatient populations in order to maintain the bottom line while enhancing the quality of care throughout the expanding continuum. Such lofty ambitions can be achieved by closely integrating services in all settings and by using case managers, both internal and external, to plan the discharge and transfer of patients.

The Home Care Example

One of the strongest forces at work stretching the continuum of care, home health services are a prime example of successful service line integration. With more programs — both freestanding and hospital-based — serving more communities, and with the recent introduction of affordable, portable technologies such as dialysis units and ventilators, almost any patient can receive appropriate services at home. The cost of home care usually is a mere fraction of the cost of a hospital stay, and many home care clients are more at ease in familiar surroundings where they can enjoy the support of family and neighbors.

The growth of home care has been built on the relationship between hospital discharge planners and home care case managers. Home care case managers can capture important client information and share in the discharge planning process by attending hospital discharge planning rounds. Sometimes, though, it is not economically feasible or cost-effective for case managers who are also clinical caregivers (nurses or therapists) to leave the field to attend hospital discharge planning rounds. Inpatient and outpatient care planners who cannot meet face-to-face must somehow establish a structure that allows a comparable exchange of information.

In referring an inpatient to home care, the home care agency should receive all pertinent patient information as early as possible in the course of acute treatment so that an appropriate case manager can be assigned. Shared data should include at least the following:

- A medical history
- Physical symptoms
- Financial information
- Psychosocial issues that may affect or delay discharge
- Family support systems (closest relative)

With this information, the home care case manager is better able to assist in discharge planning and better prepared to allocate home care resources wisely.

For example, an elderly orthopedic patient who had elective surgery and an uncomplicated course of treatment at the hospital may require only routine follow-up care. However, if the patient required emergency hip surgery, lives alone, and has no family support system, planning for home care can become rather complex. When the patient is admitted to the nursing unit, information obtained from the patient or a family member can be directed to discharge planners or transmitted to the social services or home care department. Having received this initial information, the home care case manager is able to plan a course of care that considers the client's individualized needs, the availability of support systems, and finances. Acting on continuous updates from the discharge planner regarding the client's progress, on the day of discharge the case manager dispatches the appropriate home care personnel, such as a physical therapist or home care aide, and any special equipment or supplies. By the time the patient is ready to leave, a walker is delivered to the hospital for the trip home and transportation arrangements have already been coordinated.

Other Examples

The plan would be about the same for the transfer of a patient requiring extended acute care to a skilled care, rehabilitation, or nursing home facility. However, regional shortages of beds for certain patient types may limit access to the appropriate facility. For example, a patient who at the last minute is declared ineligible for home care due to a lack of support systems, but who is otherwise stable, may have to be admitted to a facility many miles from home because it is the closest one that offers a certain type of care and has an open bed on such late notice. Early evaluation and notification of social services and discharge planning staff may prevent such last-minute searches and thus enhance patient movement through the continuum.

Any strategy that bridges two or more care delivery systems without significantly increasing costs should be explored. In the pediatric program at the Pediatric Center for Restorative Care, in Dallas, nurses and therapists rotate between inpatient acute and home care settings. The nurse or therapist who cares for the child and family in the hospital follows the case into the home to ensure that teaching plans and other goals established by the inpatient program are completed. Although staffing and time scheduling have posed some challenges, the concept has been enthusiastically accepted by physicians, patients, families, and staff. There currently is insufficient data to gauge the broader applicability of Baylor's approach, but it certainly works well for the center's population.

Regardless of the services or their setting, an organized system of predischarge planning and advance notification of agencies is an absolute requirement for any health care provider wishing to achieve a continuum of care.

• The Comprehensive Plan of Care

The individual patient care plan developed in the hospital offers valuable information to home care case managers and other allied health providers. It is the people who establish and supervise the inpatient care plan who are the best hope for informed planning of postdischarge services.

Physician education is most helpful in making a discharge plan work. Because physicians probably are in the best position to know whether their patients will require additional assistance upon discharge, they should be encouraged to write orders for social services or home health referrals early on. The patient's primary nurse also is in a good position to evaluate and request assistance. Some payer-based case managers, too, are well versed in clients' support systems prior to admission and may advise or request early discharge planning. Significant time and resources are saved when staff can be scheduled ahead of time, durable medical equipment and other supplies made available, and appropriate health care professionals and staff, such as physical therapists and home health aides, scheduled as required.

Last-minute adjustments may be required in any plan, but a seamless continuum is virtually impossible to achieve without one. Following is how a comprehensive plan of care should unfold:

- The hospital caregiver or primary nurse develops and writes the plan of care to include the entire spell of illness, not just the hospital stay, with frequent updates and modifications based on reevaluation of patient progress and complications.
- For each problem identified, the plan of care specifies a critical pathway of interventions and short- and long-term goals and outcome indicators.
- The client's progress is monitored periodically by the primary nurse, the case manager, or a multidisciplinary team, as specified in the plan, until the episode of illness is complete and the patient has achieved the goals set for both inpatient (short-term) and outpatient (long-term) care.

Figure 6-3 illustrates a comprehensive plan of care for postoperative joint replacement.

• Quality Monitors and Outcomes

The written plan of care must specify measurable outcomes. In monitoring quality of care, it is important to focus on the outcomes of the total care delivered, perhaps in several settings. The development of outcome indicators and monitoring mechanisms requires a multidisciplinary approach within the hospital or skilled facility as well as cooperation among case managers representing various agencies. Obtaining meaningful results and analyzing them must be a shared responsibility.

Figure 6-3. Plan of Care for Postoperative Joint Replacement

Date/Time ID'ed	Discipline/ Signature	Problem	Interventions	Short-Term Goals/ Outcome Indicators	Date Resolved/ Discipline	Long-Term Goals/ Outcome Indicators	Date Resolved/ Discipline

		Impaired mobility related to postop joint replacement
		a. Hip
		b. Knee
		c. Other
			1. Change position every 2 hours
			2. Support joint in alignment
			  a. In bed
			  b. In chair
			  c. When walking
			  d. During transfers
			3. Perform passive range of motion as ordered
			4. Use appliances as ordered
			  a. TEDs
			  b. CPM
			  c. Splints
			  d. Abduction pillow
			  e. Walker
			  f. Cane
				1. Patient will be able to bear weight on replaced joint for ____ minutes
				2. Patient will be able to walk ____ feet
				  a. With assist
				  b. Without assist
				3. Patient will obtain
				  ____ Degree flexion
				  ____ Degree extension
				  ____ Extension lag
						1. Patient will be able to walk ____ feet within ____ weeks
						  a. With assist
						  b. Without assist
						2. Patient will be able to
						  a. Manage steps in and out of home
						  b. Transfer to car
						  c. ____
						  d. ____
						  e. ____
						3. Patient will obtain
						  ____ Degree flexion
						  ____ Degree extension
						  ____ Extension lag
						4. Patient will be able to perform home exercise routine
						  a. Independently
						  b. With cuing
						  c. With minimal assist	

Date/Time ID'ed	Discipline/ Signature	Problem	Interventions	Short-Term Goals/ Outcome Indicators	Date Resolved/ Discipline	Long-Term Goals/ Outcome Indicators	Date Resolved/ Discipline

		Risk of postoperative complications
		a. Infection
		b. Skin breakdown
		c. Neurovascular changes
		d. Postoperative joint instability/ dislocation
		e. Other
			1. Assess incision for
			  a. Signs of infection
			  b. Healing vs. breakdown
			2. Monitor temperature
			3. Assess skin for
			  a. Redness
			  b. Edema
			  c. _____
			4. Assess neurovascular status
			  a. Numbness
			  b. Tingling
			  c. Color/temperature change
			5. Turn to unaffected side only
			6. Maintain correct position
			  a. In bed
			  b. In chair
			  c. When walking
			  d. During transfers
			7. Report to physician
			  a. Signs of infection
			  b. Neurologic changes
			  c. Patient noncompliance with activity restrictions
			  d. _____
				1. Patient will have incision healed at time of discharge
				2. Patient will not develop skin breakdown
				3. Patient will not develop joint dislocation
						1. Suture line will be healed	

(Continued on next page)

Figure 6-3. (Continued)

Date/Time ID'ed	Discipline/ Signature	Problem	Interventions	Short-Term Goals/ Outcome Indicators	Date Resolved/ Discipline	Long-Term Goals/ Outcome Indicators	Date Resolved/ Discipline
		Knowledge deficit concerning a. Safety issues b. When to call doctor c. Postoperative self-care	1. Teach patient/caregiver a. Signs of infection b. To report changes in sensation or color c. ROM exercises d. Proper positioning e. Activity restrictions f. _____ g. _____ 2. Consider referrals for a. Home care b. Home equipment c. _____ 3. Assess environment for a. Safety b. Barriers c. _____ d. _____	1. Patient/caregiver will be able to state when to call the doctor 2. Patient/caregiver will be able to perform ROM exercises a. Independently b. With supervision 3. Patient/caregiver will be able to state post-discharge services/ appointments		1. Patient/caregiver will be able to state a. When to call doctor b. Safety measure to take at home c. Emergency measures taught d. _____ e. _____ f. _____	

Several elements may be used to develop measurable outcome indicators. These include:

- Functional goals for patient or caregiver
- Teaching/learning self-care skills
- Patient's/caregiver's ability, both physically and mentally, to perform needed skills
- Ability, both financial and physical, to obtain needed supplies, equipment, or services
- Patient/caregiver satisfaction with services
- Cost
- Cohesiveness of service; delays, utilization review, goals met

Quality monitors help planners coordinate care by defining caregivers' roles and responsibilities in achieving maximum patient outcomes.

• Financial Considerations

One of the challenges of working in a large decentralized system is coming to grips with the emphasis on financial information at the department level. Although that is important, total emphasis on departmental finances also is the leading cause of turf battles between departments that should be working together.

For example, a discharged orthopedic patient may be eligible for both home care service and outpatient therapy from the physical medicine department. Realistically, either department could meet the patient's needs. But even with objective intent, the emphasis on departmental finances urges each department to focus on increasing its own revenues. The fervent cry today, particularly with the imminent movement toward one payment for the entire span of care, is to choose the types of services that best suit the patient's needs and are the most cost-effective for the system. Total product line control and costing of services, an organizational structure that has been used successfully by some smaller hospitals and by many HMOs, may be one answer.

How Product Line Management Works

Returning to the earlier example of the total hip replacement patient whose needs could be met by either home care or outpatient therapy, the discharge planning process at Baylor employs an orthopedic case manager who coordinates all postdischarge patient care and, depending on the patient's assessed needs, would contract with either home care or outpatient therapy. The discharge plan of care is further developed by a multidisciplinary team based in the orthopedic department. Even though the plan of care is coordinated by the orthopedic case manager, the administrative, management, staffing, licensure, and maintenance standards are handled by the departmental management team. Similar systems could be used for other hospital product lines — cardiovascular, oncology, wound care, and so on. A diagram of the organizational structure of such a system is shown in figure 6-4.

The concept of service departments subcontracting for product line management can position the system for the advent of managed care, which is penetrating most health care markets. Managed care organizations are looking for service packages that provide cost-effective, high-quality service. Serving both inpatient and outpatient populations, hospital-based systems are uniquely prepared to combine all program components in a single package and to offer and contract services for personalized plans of care.

How Product Line Management Contains Costs

The following is how a cost-effective personalized plan of care can be developed for the example patient admitted to the hospital orthopedic unit for a total hip replacement. The hospital has a contract with the payer, an HMO, to pay a given dollar amount. The challenge for the hospital is to provide excellent care for the patient without allowing the expenses to exceed that dollar amount. The orthopedic product line assigns a case manager, who arranges with the surgery department to replace the hip at a preagreed cost. Thus, surgery becomes a cost rather than a revenue center. The patient then spends three to eight days on the nursing unit at a cost of approximately $600 per day, excluding hospital and system overhead costs. Any therapy, physical or occupational, is provided at cost by the physical medicine department and is not entered as revenue by that department. Following therapy, the orthopedic case manager contracts for postdischarge services with another cost center, such as a skilled nursing facility, a home care agency, or the outpatient physical medicine department.

It is essential that each patient's care be managed separately and provided in the environment that best meets his or her needs. In this case, the plan of care is determined by the orthopedic product line case manager in collaboration with the primary physician. Coordinating the plan and communicating with providers to update the plan so that it continues to meet the patient's needs is the responsibility of the case manager.

As physicians have become more knowledgeable about health care issues, care continuums, and costs, they have become the key members of the planning team. Because they ultimately are responsible for the patient's medical management, physicians' preferences and directives normally reign. Thus, physician support of the care continuum and case management package is paramount to its success. In the successful case management system, the case manager knows and includes the primary physician in the core development of the plan of care.

Figure 6-4. Organizational Structure for Total Product Line Control and Costing of Services

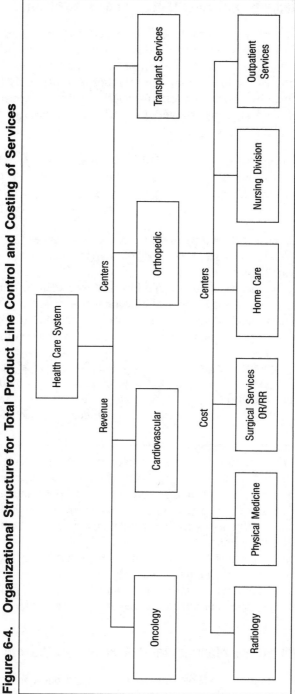

Reprinted, with permission, from Baylor Center for Restorative Care, Dallas, TX, copyright 1993.

• Case Management Alternatives and Responsibilities

What options are available to the case manager? Depending on their age and physical condition, different patients may be candidates for different combinations of care. A 62-year-old patient with a hip fracture but no other significant physical problems may leave the hospital after only five days, receive treatment by a home care team for another week, and possibly return to outpatient physical therapy for additional treatment as needed, with costs as follows:

Acute inpatient days	5 days @ $600	$3,000
Home care visits	6 visits @ $85	510
Outpatient therapy	5 visits @ $60	300
	Total cost	$3,810

If a package price of $6,000 has been negotiated in advance for the whole procedure, the system is left with a $2,200 margin to cover any overhead or unanticipated costs.

On the other hand, an 80-year-old hip fracture patient with hypertension and heart disease may stay in the hospital five or six days and then be transferred to a skilled nursing facility (SNF) for another 10 days before going home for 10 more home care therapy visits, with costs as follows:

Acute inpatient days	9 days @ $600	$5,400
SNF days	10 days @ $300	3,000
Home care visits	10 visits @ $85	850
	Total cost	$9,250

The negotiated package price for this client may be $8,000 to $10,000. Currently, the three care providers here may have very different reimbursement systems for this Medicare client: the hospital on a fixed payment system, the SNF on a combination of fixed and cost-based, and the home care agency on cost-based with caps on certain services. Each provider needs to analyze its own reimbursement issues so that the patient's needs can be met in the most cost-effective manner.

A good care plan must make good sense. Sound case management recognizes that each patient is a human being with special clinical and psychosocial needs. The resources utilized by patients will vary widely, depending on the support systems and resources they need to get well.

• Outpatient Case Management: A Focus on the Future

Alternative settings are no longer alternative. With a burgeoning ambulatory care industry and rapidly changing demographics, there are now more client service needs in the outpatient care environment, making ambulatory care the primary market for case management services. Hospitals may remain the hubs of our health care system, but they may not always be the prime movers in the continuum. Strategic plans and contracting arrangements will have to make room for case management programs developed by and designed for facilities other than acute care hospitals and systems. New forces and new combinations of forces are already at work.

Two associated outpatient programs — for example, an outpatient surgery center and a home care agency — can develop packages that include both procedures and follow-up care to meet the specific needs of patients and payers. For example, a 38-year-old client undergoing a vaginal hysterectomy at an ambulatory surgery center might generate the following costs:

Surgical procedure	$1,350
Private duty nurse/LVN (60 hours)	810
Follow-up RN visits (3)	210
Personal care aide (4 hours × 3 days)	144
Supplies	45
Medications/IVs	95
Miscellaneous	50
Total cost	$2,704

If the ambulatory surgery center negotiated a package price of $3,200 for this client, its margin to cover overhead would be $500. But it is risky to negotiate package prices without knowing costs. Here, the exact costs will vary with the number of private duty hours and registered nurse visits as well as with the amounts of medications and supplies needed. Once the costs associated with a procedure are firmly established, reimbursement rates can be negotiated with third-party payers.

The administrators of the outpatient surgery component might market the program, negotiate with the payer, add in the average cost of providing care in the home, schedule and monitor the continuum of care, and send one bill for all care components to the payer. Or, home care services might be provided at cost to the outpatient surgery center in an integrated system or with a marginal profit for independent agents. In this case, home care becomes a cost center for the case management program developed by the outpatient surgery center. Administrative billing and management overhead would be included in the cost of home care visits, though marketing, billing procedures, and bad debt might not be incorporated in direct costing applications.

• Conclusion

Case management holds the key to the continuum of care that has eluded so many providers. Whether developed and run by members of an integrated health care system or by an independent organization, case management programs can align a vast array of distinct resources into a whole that is at once comprehensive and comprehensible. A coordinated continuum of care for patients sometimes lost in the shuffle, a cost-effective product for payers demanding one, a convincing answer for health care organizations with strong community missions but strapped for cash — any program that can deliver on such promises is sure to be a major component of future health care delivery.

Bibliography

Brueckner, G., and Frasca, C. Integrating home care into hospital/ambulatory care delivery systems. *Outreach* 13(3):1,3, May–June 1992.

Evashwick, C., and Weiss, L., editors. *Managing the Continuum of Care.* Rockville, MD: Aspen Publishers, 1987.

Knollmueller, R. N. Case management: what's in a name? *Nursing Management* 20(10):38–42, Oct. 1989.

Matheis-Kraft, C., George, S., Olinger, M. J., and York, L. Patient-driven healthcare works! *Nursing Management* 21(9):124, 125, 128, Sept. 1990.

O'Malley, J., Loveridge, C. E., and Cummings, S. H. The new nursing organization. *Nursing Management* 20(2):29–32, Feb. 1989.

Pierog, L. J. Case management: a product line. *Nursing Administration Quarterly* 15(2):16–20, Winter 1991.

Warner-Handelsman, J. The home care contribution to continuity of care. *Nursing Administration Quarterly* 15(4):61–64, Summer 1991.

Weiss, L. J. A care coordination system: relief for overwhelmed patients. *Continuing Care* 7(10):29–31, Oct. 1988.

Chapter 7

The Caregiver as Case Manager

Dawn Lajeunesse

• Introduction

It is widely acknowledged that physicians and allied health professionals are the best-qualified care managers and should therefore be granted ultimate authority for the medical management of their patients. However, patients and families today present a diversity of complex clinical, environmental, and social needs that defy traditional notions of medical management. Confronted with a dizzying selection of treatment and referral options, health care providers are just now learning how to coordinate the healing process in its entirety, in all settings, case by case. Among the strongest case management programs are those that recognize the central role of primary caregivers in serving clients' individual health and social needs without neglecting the cost of care. Many are finding that the patient bedside still offers the best vantage point for coordinating clinically efficacious and cost-effective health care.

The case management process goes well beyond mere medical management. A good case manager is a care coordinator in the largest sense — facilitating access to a continuum of medical and social services, planning courses of treatment in a variety of settings, and allocating resources according to the individual needs of patients and their families. Unfortunately, in today's fragmented health care system, assignment of a case manager is often left to chance. A client's point of entry or referral — though often more a matter of circumstance than an indicator of need or appropriate treatment — determines whether his or her case manager will be a nurse, a social worker, a physical therapist, a counselor, or some other professional or paraprofessional.

Part of this chapter is based on the following article: D. A. Lajeunesse. Case management: a primary nursing approach. *Caring* 9(8):13–16, Aug. 1990. Used, with permission, from the National Association for Home Care.

Because assignment of the best-qualified case manager is so crucial to ensuring high-quality patient care across the continuum, providers cannot take this responsibility lightly. Organizations that aspire to provide comprehensive case management must first choose the most suitable care coordinator who can best help clients access the services and resources they need, while keeping an eye on costs. Only then can the organization proceed to implement an effective case management process that clients and caregivers will follow with confidence and ease.

This chapter discusses how care management of a changing outpatient population is necessitating greater coordination and provides an illustration of how to set up case manager responsibilities using the experience of the Visiting Nurse Service Association of Schenectady County in Schenectady, New York. It also describes how the nursing model of case management differs from the traditional nursing process and how the cost control function might be incorporated in the care management program design.

• Coordinating Outpatient Care for a Changing Population

In the past decade, the outpatient population has not only grown, but it has become more diverse. As a result, the case management needs of this population have become more complex, requiring greater coordination in the provision of care and the determination of appropriate resources. Ideally, that case management responsibility would be undertaken by a single caregiver.

The Care-Giving Case Manager

In the home health care industry and among leaders in professional nursing, there is an educated bias that caregivers make the best case managers. Proponents of caregiver case management feel that adding a layer to the health care system for the sole purpose of coordinating services causes unnecessary expense and a wasteful duplication of effort. Studies show that when the clinical assessment function is separated from the case management function, caregivers become confused, patient care is delayed, and services are duplicated. A single service provider, with the help of fellow caregivers and widely understood screening and monitoring processes, can handle both the assessment and case management functions more efficiently.[1]

As home health care is no longer focused primarily on the elderly but serves a diverse population of acute and chronically ill children and adults, the Area Agencies on Aging should not be expected to function as the general point of entry into the home care delivery system. Because of the trend to move all patients out of the hospital rapidly, or not to admit them in the first place, the home care delivery system is administering the care and case management needs of a population of all ages — from newborns and pediatric patients, to adolescents, to young and middle-aged adults, and particularly the elderly.

Deploying the Right Resources

No one knows the patient/consumer as well as the provider, and service provision should, after all, be customer-driven as well as financially driven. Further, not everyone who enters the health care delivery system needs intensive, comprehensive case management services. A patient requiring a single service of short duration does not require the same coordinated effort as someone requiring services from multiple disciplines, community agencies, and clinics. The professional provider has the expertise to recognize the difference and to adjust or combine resources appropriately to avoid more costly services than the patient actually needs. Case management also affords the opportunity to provide the emotional support so important to clients in today's sometimes impersonal health care system.

The Long-Term Home Health Care Program in New York State is a shining example of provider health and social service agencies working cooperatively to manage costs and meet a broad range of needs for a broad range of clients. Essentially, the program is a "nursing home without walls" that serves clients of all ages, not just the elderly. By coordinating the provision of long-term care services in the familiar comfort of the client's own home, the Long-Term Home Health Care Program makes wise use of expensive specialized resources by involving family, friends, and the clients themselves in the daily care routine. Without the program, these individuals would require more costly and less desirable institutional services.

The Value of One Good Case Manager

Often several case management efforts must be coordinated to avoid duplication of services. For example, it is not unusual for an oncology patient to be receiving services both in an outpatient oncology clinic and at home through a certified home health agency. The same patient may be receiving homemaker or personal care services under the direction of the local social services department or the Office for Aging. And, of course, the patient's requirements may change, obviating the need for some services and adding others, such as hospice.

Ideally, one centrally located, highly trained, and well-regarded case manager should coordinate the multiple services and sources of reimbursement, maintaining frequent communication with all involved entities. In the outpatient setting, this case manager must be particularly knowledgeable of clinical, fiscal, social, and community resources. A knowledgeable case manager is the essential link in providing assessments and interventions that match resources with consumer needs. Looking beyond the paradigms to choose the best, safest, and most financially acceptable matrix of required services requires considerable time, energy, and creativity.

But sound case management is not an automatic function, and program success will surely vary with case managers' levels of education and training, the program's geographic scope, and the availability of resources in the region. It is all the more important, then, that core program attributes — knowledgeable case managers and a reliable network of resources — be cultivated and supported by the sponsoring case management, home health care, or human service agency or employer. Long-range program goals also should include the continuing education of physicians, nurses, therapists, and social workers to maintain a fresh supply of trained case managers.

• Establishing Case Management Responsibilities

Selecting the case manager most suitable for the client population is the first and perhaps most crucial step in establishing an effective case management program. The case manager is the personality and character of the program and, ultimately, makes or breaks it. The case manager must command knowledge, collegial respect, and clout in the program's circle of nurses, referring physicians, and contracted providers. Thus, this most important of positions must be filled carefully and defined clearly.

The experience of the Visiting Nurse Service Association of Schenectady County (VNSA), a home health agency, illustrates the establishment of case manager responsibilities in three steps: role definition, client referral, and case manager assignment. The following subsections describe those steps.

The Role of Case Manager

At VNSA, the primary care nurse (PCN) most frequently is the acknowledged case manager, although a physical or speech therapist may assume the role if nursing care is not required. The role of case manager has evolved and its scope expanded due to higher patient acuity levels as well as changing state and federal regulations. The early discharge of patients from hospitals has provided the opportunity and necessity for primary nurse case managers to be proactive in assessing patients' needs at home and advocating on their behalf to obtain the care and services they require in their recovery. Primary nurse case management in home care must take a holistic, not a task-oriented approach to care. Four years ago, drawing on this author's experience in another agency, the VNSA more formally defined the scope and concept of the PCN's case management responsibilities.

Because the VNSA case manager usually is a primary care nurse, the case management process is formally modeled after the nursing process. The nursing process lends the case management program a familiar, logical organization and sequence of activities, as described in detail later in this chapter.

In short, the case manager is the professional responsible for overseeing all of the patient's fundamental needs. As mentioned above, the approach is holistic. The nurse assesses the needs of the total patient, not an isolated symptom or task, and includes the family and environment, as they may affect the patient's care needs. She or he plays matchmaker, assessing where the patient and family are on a continuum of functioning, and links them with an appropriate array of formal and informal community services. The case manager coordinates all of those services and disciplines and intervenes to make adjustments when care needs change. She or he also anticipates and plans for discharge from agency services, making sure that any remaining needs are managed through an alternate resource.

The case manager may change as the patient's primary needs change. For example, a primary care nurse may transfer case management responsibilities to a physical therapist as a rehabilitation client's condition improves and the primary caregiver relationship shifts from nurse to therapist. In multidisciplinary programs, identity of the primary case manager should be conspicuously documented and every change of case managers should be broadcast to other departments or agencies immediately.

The Referral Process

The VNSA case management program swings into action as soon as the client is referred to the home health agency by a hospital discharge planner, physician, family member, or other referral source. Seasoned community health nurses functioning as liaisons in local hospitals ask the discharge planner or physician probing questions about the patient's specific needs and make recommendations for meeting those needs in the home care system. Calls coming into the agency directly are filtered through an intake supervisor, also an experienced community health nurse, who plays a parallel role in the quality assurance program. This ensures that the patient is entered into an active quality assessment process before services are even implemented. The intake supervisor sorts through the information provided by the referral source, asks for more details where needed, and makes some preliminary assessments about the patient's care needs, including:

- Disciplines that may be required to provide care
- The estimated frequency and duration of services
- The need for and nature of physician involvement
- Diagnoses that may affect care planning
- The need to involve other community services
- Supplies and equipment needed

- Any referrals already made to other resources
- The availability of third-party payers and the eligibility of services for payment
- Other financial resources that may need to be considered
- Family and other informal support systems

This initial assessment is merely preliminary to the in-home comprehensive assessment later conducted by the PCN. However, the intake supervisor's assessment does provide the PCN some guidance in establishing an approach and making preparations for the initial visit, and it minimizes surprises and maximizes the effectiveness of the PCN's or admitting nurse's time. It further assures the patient that caregivers are talking to each other and working together.

Case Manager Assignment

Once a patient has entered the home health agency's care delivery system, a PCN/case manager is assigned. Usually geography plays a key role in the selection of the case manager, because limiting travel time and distance is integral to containing the cost of services. Specialized skills, such as infusion therapy certification or pediatric expertise, also may need to be considered. Various specialty areas are represented on each nursing team, and the team supervisor presently makes the final assignment decisions. (The VNSA has been transitioning to a total quality management model since early 1992. It is presumed that, eventually, the individual teams will be self-directing and functionally autonomous in case manager assignment and cost control.)

All patients are seen by a case manager within 24 hours of referral unless specifically requested for later, and many, depending on their need, are admitted to the program the same day. Strictly speaking, the case management process begins the moment the client is admitted to the program.

• Applying the Nursing Model of Case Management

The five phases of the traditional nursing process — assessment, diagnosis, planning, implementation, and evaluation — provide a conveniently familiar and effective framework for nurse-directed case management. In the nursing model of case management, the five phases become seven:

1. Patient and family assessment
2. Problem identification
3. Care planning
4. Delegation of care responsibilities

5. Intervention
6. Coordination and collaboration of disciplines
7. Evaluation of outcomes

The case management process is slightly altered and expanded because, beyond coordinating the client's care, the case manager also is responsible for coordinating reimbursement, including assessing payer sources, anticipating changes in clients' courses of treatment and their impact, planning for those changes, and providing the documentation necessary to support reimbursement. Figure 7-1 shows how the case management process parallels the traditional nursing process.

Patient and Family Assessment

Complete client physical, psychosocial, and environmental data are obtained in a thorough initial assessment. This assessment may cover, but is not limited to, household members and their relationship to the patient, environmental factors that might affect the patient's well-being (running water, cleanliness, bugs, heating, and so on), family dynamics, financial resources, community supports, and all physicians involved in serving the patient's health care needs. The case manager identifies the patient's preepisodic level of functioning (without which goals may be set unrealistically) and performs a complete physical assessment to define the current baseline status.

Assessments are repeated periodically while the patient is on the caseload, allowing the case manager to evaluate the need for intervention by other disciplines or community resources. In the assessment phase, the case manager also begins to determine the most appropriate source of reimbursement for services and formulates preliminary estimates of the frequency and duration of services that will be required to return the patient and family to the highest reasonable level of self-care.

Figure 7-1. The Nursing and Case Management Processes Compared

Traditional Nursing Process	Case Management Process
Assessment	Patient and family assessment
Diagnosis	Problem identification
Planning	Care planning
Implementation	Delegation of care responsibilities Intervention Coordination/collaboration of disciplines
Evaluation	Evaluation of outcomes

Problem Identification

Using the data obtained during assessment, the case manager establishes nursing diagnoses and identifies the problems to be addressed in the care plan. The diagnoses should include the psychosocial factors that may affect the patient's recovery, such as a history of noncompliance, ineffective coping, lack of knowledge, lack of motivation, or other family stressors. The case manager identifies present and potential problems as well as managed problems that do not require agency intervention. In the latter case, documentation should indicate how and when the problem is managed and by whom. A thorough case manager will observe the care that is being provided by an informal caregiver. For example, if a patient's daily insulin injections are administered by a neighbor, the nurse case manager should observe the neighbor's procedure to ensure correct and safe technique.

Care Planning

The next step in the case management process is development of an individualized and comprehensive plan of care. *Individualized* means that, for example, if a patient requires sliding insulin doses, the specific blood sugar parameters that govern the dosage should be noted in the care plan. Goals need to be specific, patient-centered, realistic, and measurable if the caregiver is to have objective data on which to base an evaluation of outcomes.

Goals should be established with the patient's/family's input and should include discussion and planning for the patient's discharge. Patients and families should understand from the initiation of services that the agency is working to achieve the patient's independence for a safe discharge and that it is not the agency's (or the payer's) intent to extend a case indefinitely. If care will be needed for extended periods, every effort should be made to teach the patient or family how to perform a treatment or provide care. A patient or family in a financial position to pay privately for continuing services may elect that option, and the agency may elect to comply. But it usually is in the patient's best interest to discourage dependence on formal caregivers as much as possible.

Case managers have an obligation to third-party payers to reduce the frequency and limit the duration of services without jeopardizing the provision of high-quality, professional care that fully meets patients' needs. In the absence of someone who can be taught to assume the patient's care safely and dependably, though, the agency has an obligation to continue care as long as there is a medical and/or nursing need.

The case manager is responsible for ongoing review and revision of the plan of care. The plan should be reviewed at least every 60 days but must be updated immediately whenever new problems are identified, new treatments are prescribed, new physician orders are received, community resources change, or goals are achieved.

Delegation of Care Responsibilities

Primary nurse case managers usually can provide the skilled nursing care for all their clients, but large caseloads, time off, and the appropriate utilization of other levels of care frequently may require the PCN to delegate responsibilities and instruct or supervise other personnel. Other nursing professionals (per diem registered nurses (RNs) or other staff RNs) who cover for the case manager are responsible for following up on any needs identified during their coverage, including obtaining supplemental orders, revising the care plan, and making appropriate phone calls. Any action taken is, of course, documented, but the replacement nurse should call attention to the action by leaving a note or verbal message for the case manager. Still, the primary nurse bears ultimate responsibility for maintaining the patient record and following up on care needs.

When a paraprofessional is involved in a case, the case manager orients, instructs, and supervises him or her and documents these activities in the patient record. The contribution that a paraprofessional worker can make in an interdisciplinary team conference should not be underestimated, and the case manager, in delegating responsibilities and in less formal situations, should communicate with paraprofessionals and encourage their participation.

In order to ensure continuity of patient care, especially in the case manager's absence, the case manager should perform certain routine tasks. These include:

- Keep the patient visit calendar up-to-date so that planned visits are not missed
- Sign up patients for weekend or holiday visits as early as the need is known, to assist in planning for staffing on those days
- Notify the on-call nurse if a visit is needed during hours when there are no regular staff on duty
- Make requests for evening visits as early as possible
- Communicate with peers for patient coverage on days off
- Make sure that the patient record is available for associates when needed

The case manager's additional responsibilities and professional obligations include providing opportunities for associates to learn new or infrequently used nursing skills. The case manager should conduct demonstrations for less experienced staff and instruct them when their patients require such skills. The case manager also is obligated to participate in team discussion to ensure daily patient coverage (for example, identifying patients for licensed practical nurse (LPN) visits or sharing overloads from another case manager's calendar). Another important professional role is collaboration among team members to find innovative solutions for patient problems that are resisting current approaches.

Intervention

In a primary nursing approach to case management, direct patient care and documentation of that care are integral parts of the case manager's role. The treatments performed by the primary care nurse may, after a period of instruction, be taken over by a family member, informal caregiver, or the patient.

In the assessment phase, the case manager identifies the availability of caregivers and gauges their ability, knowledge, and technical skill levels. In the intervention phase, the case manager instructs the patient and/or caregiver in specific skills and informs them about the disease process, applicable medications, and so on. Instruction should include demonstrations by the nurse and return demonstrations by the patient or caregiver. In documenting teaching activities and outcomes, the case manager might write, for example, "patient able to list signs and symptoms" or "wife performed complete dressing change correctly." The documentation also may note the patient's inability to perform self-treatment safely and/or the lack of a competent caregiver for instruction.

Contacting and coordinating assistance with other disciplines and with community resources plays an important role in the intervention step. The timely and appropriate utilization of such services as Meals-on-Wheels, special transportation, or adult day care distinguishes a successful home care plan that meets its patients' total care needs.

The case manager reviews the patient's status on a continuous basis, identifying changes requiring reinstruction. For example, a wound care treatment may be modified if it is deemed less effective than desired. The patient and/or caregiver would then have to be instructed in the new procedure. Or, if a patient's primary caregiver becomes unavailable due to hospitalization or for some other reason, another caregiver would need to be trained.

One particularly sensitive responsibility of the case manager involves realistically evaluating the client's progress and long-range expectations, and activating other mechanisms to provide care as needed. For example, the time may come for a patient with a terminal illness to be offered the option of hospice services. Likewise, a patient with a degenerative condition or an increasingly frail caregiver may need to be told to consider planning for long-term options such as nursing home placement. It usually falls to the case manager, who is familiar enough with the client's total picture and trusted enough by the family, to broach such subjects. When existing interventions are not meeting goals, the case manager should initiate consults with peers, a supervisor, or the clinical nurse specialist, if the agency has one.

Coordination and Collaboration of Disciplines

Frequently, a client will require the services of multiple disciplines. In the assessment phase, the case manager initiates any necessary referrals for evaluation by other disciplines and documents them in the patient record. If there was no order for such an evaluation on the initial physician referral, the case manager should contact the physician for supplemental orders and authorization.

For the case management process to function cohesively, certain courtesies and standards of communication should be observed by all disciplines involved. These include:

- Notifying other disciplines of the hospitalization or death of a shared patient
- Coordinating visits to avoid multiple professionals visiting at the same time or overtiring the patient
- Integrating services to provide maximum benefit to the patient
- Problem solving jointly when appropriate, sharing information informally as well as in formal multidisciplinary team conferences
- Notifying other disciplines of the plan to discharge a patient
- Documenting all interactions with other disciplines, including the content and outcome of conferences, in the patient record

It also is essential to maintain close contact with community resources, to regularly review their effectiveness in meeting patients' needs, and to clarify their respective roles in order to avoid service duplication or gaps.

Evaluation of Outcomes

Perhaps no step in the case management process is as important as the evaluation of outcomes, for without careful and proper confirmation that care is proceeding as planned, the entire process may be rendered futile. Evaluation is an ongoing process, and target outcomes should be based on patient care goals established in the plan of care.

The case manager continuously reviews and assesses all aspects of care provided to ensure that the care plan is being followed effectively, that goals have been or are being achieved, and that the agency quality of care standards are met. If goals are not or cannot be accomplished, the case is reassessed and adjustments are made in the plan of care. Ultimately, anyone comparing the care plan to the patient's actual progress at various stages should be able to tell that the patient's goals are being met or that an obstacle was identified and the care plan amended to overcome that obstacle. If outcomes do not match goals, the reasons should be clear, as should appropriate follow-up actions. If standards of care are not met, the agency should have a mechanism for further review, such as discussion with the supervisor or clinical specialist or consultation with a representative of the quality assurance committee.

When all the outcomes prescribed in the care plan have been accomplished, the patient is discharged. The case manager is responsible for notifying the patient/family, physician, and other disciplines and involved community resources of the intent to discharge, and for documenting these communications. The case manager then prepares a discharge summary describing referrals made, recommendations given, and the reason for discharge.

• Including the Financial Perspective in the Case Management Process

Many payers, including the government, increasingly view case management as a separate reimbursement entity. For them, the promise of case management is not only to coordinate multiple resources for a patient's care needs, but also to assess and control the amount of care needed from a financial management perspective. Properly designed, any case management program can readily fulfill both the care and cost control roles, as many already do.

An effective program design creates a flexible scheme for handling and financing referrals from external sources as well as transfers within the program. For patients referred for medical needs, primary care nurses can provide skilled care at the standard reimbursement rate and case management (which they provide anyway) for a separate fee, at a negotiated add-on rate, or by some other arranged mechanism of reimbursement. A separate track of referrals to the case management program could be developed for clients initially referred for supportive or social services. These clients could be assigned to an agency social worker for case management. Should one of these clients develop the need for medical service, the transition to PCN case management would be easy for the client and family, because the transfer would take place, essentially, between highly cooperative departments of a single organization. The program would merely supplement existing social and support services with medical services to meet the new needs. Figure 7-2 shows how the case management program can accommodate clients' specific needs via referrals and transfers between separate but integrated medical and social service tracks.

To support these reimbursement initiatives, a clear, standardized definition of what is included in case management and objective measures of the cost of case management in provider settings must be developed and tested. These definitions and measures will demonstrate the cost-effectiveness of case management as well as provide a foundation for a controlled but reasonable reimbursement system for case management services. Among payers and business and community leaders, the most generally accepted components of case management include:[2]

- Determining eligibility for admission — financial, medical, or other
- Assessing required levels of care
- Defining specific client needs
- Assigning the site of care

- Developing care plans
- Prescribing or arranging services
- Coordinating services from multiple providers
- Budget planning for service units, duration, and episodes of care
- Reassessing needs
- Monitoring service delivery and quality
- Supporting families

These program attributes should be highlighted in any dealings with payers or other parties who must be convinced that case management is both clinically efficacious and financially sound.

The involvement of the case management program will vary with the complexity of a client's care needs. A given case manager's caseload may range from clients who simply need a single service to those requiring the coordination of multiple services and providers, changing needs, and family support and care giving. A well-designed program, with caregivers as case managers, has the ability to increase or decrease services according to need, without disruption during transfers or cross-referrals. And even if services move from nonmedical and nonskilled to multiple skilled care services, or vice versa, a program run by caregivers will likely cost less than a separately administered case management organization.

Figure 7-2. Case Management Referral and Transfer Tracks

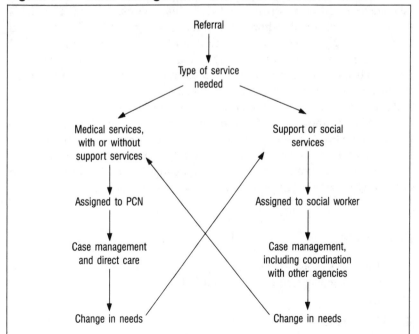

Other creative applications of payment need to be considered and studied further. Various demonstration projects nationwide have shown that case management costs can range from $49 to $145 per client per month.[3] Because case management needs vary from client to client and for individual clients over time, lump-sum grants for all case management services for a defined contract period, or an average total per case (capitation rate) cost, might be more attractive than an add-on cost per visit or a percentage of total service cost scheme. Short-term care may need to be handled differently from long-term care. A provider-based model allows the intensity of case management to ebb and flow naturally with the changes in client/family service needs. In selecting provider agencies for case management services, consideration must be given to how the agencies currently manage their costs: How do their costs compare to existing Medicare caps? What percentage of their costs goes to administration, rather than patient services?

Any payment system should include built-in disincentives for over-prescribing services, while providing assurances that clients will receive the services they genuinely need and encouraging greater efficiency in the provision of case management.

• Conclusion

There is no one best way to organize case management. Various models offer advantages in different settings and for varying needs. A nursing model is particularly well suited to home health case management, as demonstrated by the Visiting Nurse Service Association of Schenectady County.

Primary care nurses, with their comprehensive knowledge of the patient and family and their experience in coordinating services and payers, make excellent case managers. Backed up by a competent staff of RNs, therapists, and social workers, PCNs are especially adept at quickly determining patient care needs and mobilizing the resources necessary to meet those needs.

With the broad support and enthusiastic cooperation of referring physicians, payers, and business and community leaders, comprehensive case management programs staffed by primary caregivers are proliferating and expanding to serve a growing, changing outpatient population.

References

1. Williams, J. K. *Case Management: Opportunities for Service Providers.* Syracuse, NY: The Haworth Press, Inc., Feb. 25, 1992, p. iii.

2. Williams, pp. i–ii.

3. Williams, p. 23.

Part II

Chapter 8

Case Management Model: Services for the Elderly

Marcie Parker and Lawrence H. Bernstein, MD

• Introduction

Community- and family-centered case management programs for the elderly offer an excellent opportunity for hospitals to reach out to an aging population. Because it is estimated that by the year 2008 more than 25 percent of the U.S. population will be over the age of 65, a case management strategy for the elderly certainly is an idea whose time has come.[1-4]

Innovative case management programs for elderly clients and their families will be essential to all future care delivery systems. The well-designed program would couple a hospital-based case management team of geriatric care nurses and physicians with a strong outreach component that embraces the services and support provided by families, senior centers, religious organizations, social service agencies, and other community resources. The primary objectives of such a program are to empower patients and families to take part in their own course of treatment, to facilitate access to care, and to provide a full range of services for elderly clients whose needs and functional abilities vary widely.

This chapter offers ideas and discusses strategies for implementing outpatient case management programs specifically for the elderly. Managed care organizations, physicians, and hospital outpatient diagnostic and therapeutic centers can each benefit from the guidelines presented here.

• Patient Categories

The overall intent of an ideal case management program is to foster independence and enhance the quality of life for patients with modest functional losses; it is not intended to increase or fine-tune the care provided to more severely affected patients already receiving intense treatment for loss of function. Specifically, a hospital-based community geriatric program serves three patient groups:

- Patients with moderate functional loss
- Patients and families planning for future needs
- Patients and families in outright crisis

Patients with Moderate Functional Loss

A very large number of ambulatory geriatric patients live quite independently despite modest functional deficits that may require routine visits to physicians' offices, clinics, and hospital emergency departments (EDs). But even modest deficits can have an enormous potential financial and social impact for the following reasons:

- *Primary care physicians often do not recognize modest losses in functioning.* In fact, roughly 25 percent of ambulatory patients over age 65 with modest deficits in the activities of daily living, including ambulation, toileting, and self-feeding, are not recognized in primary care settings.[5]
- *Caregivers often fail to consider patients' perceptions of their own illnesses.* The patient's overall "disease burden" is greater than a sum of symptoms. For example, in the case of a patient with arthritic hands who longs to cook her own meals and dress herself, which is more important: alleviating her pain or increasing her ability to function?

Fortunately, many community resources already in place can significantly improve the quality of life for elderly patients. A diverse range of professionals such as visiting nurses, occupational and physical therapists, and others can facilitate improved functioning for patients with modest deficits in the activities of daily living. And most interventions to address modest deficits are readily available at a modest cost.

The case manager's responsibility is to recognize modest deficits and to act resourcefully to prevent further functional loss or complications. For example, a patient with a slightly unsteady gait is at great risk of falling in the shower and fracturing a hip. Virtually anyone who sees such a patient walk down a hospital corridor will notice this telltale gait. Diagnosis of a modest deficit usually does not require special expertise. The astute case manager might suggest a transfer bench for the shower, grab bars, or other inexpensive yet highly effective preventive devices and measures. Without designated nurse and physician case managers working in an organized program, health care workers in institutional settings might not notice such a modest deficit or think to suggest such a pragmatic solution.

Patients and Families Planning for Future Needs

The U.S. Census Bureau reports that the population aged 85 and older increased 232 percent between 1960 and 1990, compared to an increase of

39 percent for the total population. Projections about the size of the oldest old population when the baby boomers reach 85 are still speculative. The Census Bureau estimates that there will be about 12 million people aged 85 and older in 2040; other researchers suggest that that number could be 20 or as high as 40 million people.[6]

Not only is the population aging rapidly, but many of the new elderly are blessed with solid financial resources, higher educational attainment, and good health. More than in past generations, these elders are planning for their future, knowing that they may live 30 to 35 years past retirement. They are asking questions, looking into available resources, and planning for the time when they may gradually lose function. In all aspects of hospital-based case management, but especially in anticipatory planning for future care needs, the audience includes not only the elderly but also their adult children—the so-called sandwich generation. The hospital ought to consider the sandwich generation, with its strong and growing marketing potential, an integral part of any community-based program.

Hospitals that aspire to be leaders in community- and family-centered case management for the elderly must do a bit of anticipatory planning themselves. It is a mistake to assume that only one group of professionals should have a franchise on serving clients' anticipatory planning needs. Certainly discharge planners and case managers are central, but any of the professionals involved in caring for the elderly should be able to help clients and their families plan for future needs. There should be as many gateways to the program as there are caregivers. The successful hospital-based programs of tomorrow are taking the lead in anticipatory planning today.

Patients and Families in Outright Crisis

When families confront a medical/social crisis with an aged parent or spouse, they typically are unprepared to make critical decisions and, consequently, the family's response often is frenzied and disjointed. These families need help. More than that, they need an ombudsperson—someone to guide the family during its crisis, not just during the acute medical care.

The hospital ED is the most common site of crisis intervention for the elderly, if for no other reason than that it provides a conduit into the health care system. But for the hospital-based case management program to work, nurses and physicians must step forward to act as ombudspersons in times of family crisis. These case managers must be readily accessible, knowledgeable, and able to aggressively yet gently and compassionately guide the family in managing the crisis.

• Program Goals

There are three main goals of a hospital-based community geriatric program. These are:

1. To empower patients and families to participate in their own course of treatment
2. To facilitate access to the full continuum of clinical and social services
3. To provide some of the needed services

Achieving these goals requires a deep understanding of the elderly patient population and its unique needs.

Empowering Patients and Families

Elderly patients and their families often require assistance in articulating their health and social needs. Specific diagnostic information is important for all facets of geriatric care, but especially when decisions are urgent. The lack of any sense of diagnostic clarity makes family members feel powerless, leading them to approach problems chaotically and making it difficult for caregivers to bring the right solutions to bear.

Identifying the problem is the first step toward solving it. An informal, simple functional assessment organizes patient and family thinking so that the process of problem solving can begin. The assessment also establishes a common structure within which all team players — patient, family, informal caregivers, and health care and social services providers — can work together toward a common end. The team must establish this preliminary diagnostic construct before considering therapeutic interventions and options. An effective assessment focuses on specific functional deficits, but it does not need to be a formal evaluation process that assigns a number or a score to patients and assigns them to categories.

Within a construct that emphasizes function and provides the information clients need to understand their diagnoses and to access the appropriate services, patients and families will eagerly participate in planning and obtaining their own care. All clients must be treated as responsible partners, rather than as passive recipients of the care and services that others have decided are best. This sense of mutual responsibility and collegiality must permeate the program as a reality and not be pasted on as a thin veneer.

Facilitating Access

Once the problem has been delineated (either in great detail or preliminarily) and potential interventions are understood, the next step is to take action. For many elderly clients and their families, this is where the process comes to an abrupt halt. At some point, case managers must stop dispensing "information and referral" and start providing focused advice and guidance to help patients and families access the services, solutions, and products they need. Facilitating clients' access to the most appropriate providers is one of the chief goals of all case management efforts.

The most effective way to facilitate access to services is to speak the patient's language, which is the language of *function*. The approach to every issue must be based on the patient's functional needs. Case managers commonly make the mistake of describing potential interventions too vaguely, without regard for the patient's needs or expectations. Every description of "what is going to be done" ought to incorporate an explanation of the specific functional impact of the proposed interventions. For example, a patient who is afraid of falling on the way to the bathroom in the middle of the night might benefit from having a commode and a night-light placed in the bedroom. In addition to enabling the elderly patient to function more easily and more safely, this intervention could help him or her avoid other problems, such as soiling the bed or getting bedsores. It also may help the spouse/caregiver continue to provide care, thus avoiding institutionalization.

Providing Services

Although the hospital will be able to provide some services, most solutions are to be found in the community and in the home. Figure 8-1 presents a partial list of the many community services and resources available to elderly patients, their families, and their case managers. Duplicating existing community services, though attractive in the short run and perhaps encouraged by the hospital's marketing group, is counterproductive in the long run. Particularly as the program is getting started, it is best to think about how to

Figure 8-1. A Partial List of Community Resources for the Elderly

• Screening and prevention programs	• Intergenerational home sharing
• Congregate meals	• Homemaking services
• Senior centers	• Chore services
• Nutrition sites	• Weatherization and repair services
• Meals-on-Wheels	• Home health care
• Golden Age clubs	• Hospice care
• Support groups (stroke club, widowed persons' service, Alzheimer's and related diseases groups, cancer support groups)	• Independent living situations
	• Boarding homes
	• Residential care and assisted living centers
• Caregiver support groups	• Intermediate nursing facilities
• Family service agencies	• Skilled nursing facilities
• Area Agencies on Aging	• Rehabilitation hospitals
• State agencies for the elderly or adult protective services	• Acute care hospitals
	• Friendly visitors
• Legal Aid	• Telephone reassurance
• Mental health care and counseling	• Escort services
• Adult day care	• Senior peer counseling
• Respite care and companions	

nurture the outpatient services the hospital already provides or those that already exist in the local community.

The program's overall goal remains the same: to facilitate access to care. To be sure, clients whose needs have been clearly articulated, whose case managers have recommended solutions germane to their functional needs, and whose families have been made to feel they are active participants in the care process will use the hospital's services eventually.

• Implementation

The success of a hospital-based case management program will hinge on its acceptance by the community at large; and with a good marketing strategy, community acceptance will be easy to achieve. On the other hand, acceptance of the program by the medical community will depend on communication with primary care physicians. Program marketers and administrators must establish a dialogue with primary care physicians in a context that appeals to the physicians' clinical experience and perspective. The hospital must deliver a clear and unequivocal message: We are working with you, supporting your clinical efforts in dealing with complex family and patient care issues, and not seeking to take patients away from your practice.

Once the case management concept has won community and physician support, the program's services and interventions can be arranged through outreach efforts with senior centers, religious settings (synagogues, churches, mosques), community social service agencies, physicians' offices, clinics, and many other community health care and social service providers. Again, a focused, hospital-based functional assessment is very fruitful and can be highly cost-efficient. Even a rudimentary approach to assessing the patient's activities of daily living and instrumental activities of daily living (for example, using the telephone, shopping for food, writing checks, monitoring a budget) will aid the hospital in implementing a program that is effective from the very start. As case managers begin assessing elderly clients' functional deficits, the hospital's occupational, physical, and speech therapy departments might even receive new referrals, helping to offset the cost of program start-up.

• The Unique Needs of Elderly Clients

The dominant theme and thrust of a newly conceived case management program for the elderly ought to be that this population has different needs and perceptions and, therefore, requires programs that are different from those of other populations served by the hospital. Hospital leaders must recognize the unique needs of elderly clients in establishing a case management program and seize the opportunity to (1) reeducate themselves and the community and (2) reengineer the organization to better serve an aging population. Specifically, hospitals might do well to heed the following advice:

- Hospitals should take the lead in increasing public awareness that the elderly with modest functional loss are a shamefully neglected part of the community. Simple, cost-effective interventions can have a dramatic impact on the health of these elderly. Physician and nurse case managers should work to reduce expensive high-tech care and enhance needed low-tech care, keeping patients with modest functional loss out of the hospital when hospital care is unnecessary; at the same time, they should encourage support for family and community caregivers.
- Hospitals should consider reorienting their historical missions as centers of high-tech acute care and, instead, emphasize wellness and prevention to help elderly clients maintain dignity and independence.
- Hospitals should function as resource centers to develop or pay for community services or, at the very least, to enhance, encourage, and support existing and developing community- and family-based services. Hospitals could fulfill this role by providing staff for education and training, arranging referrals, developing a community services directory or consumer manual, or paying for joint community services advertising. The important point is to foster within the elderly community a sense of the hospital as the place to turn for services not traditionally provided in hospitals. The elderly must come to think of the hospital as a resource center and a place to receive excellent outpatient services and referrals.
- Hospitals should require all staff (physicians, nursing staff, dietitians, aides, housekeepers, and others) to learn about and appreciate the disease burden imposed by elderly chronic illness. Institution-based professionals, in particular, must be aware of long-term care and the full continuum of care. Continuing education for staff might be achieved by having members rotate one day annually through home health care, adult day care, nursing homes, Meals-on-Wheels, friendly visiting, and telephone reassurance or respite care services. Elder care rotations may be supplemented by quarterly training through appropriate videos, films, and guest lectures and role-plays about community services, long-term care, and family/informal care.
- Hospital staff should rethink their treatment of hospitalized geriatric patients and return as much control as possible to the patient and the family. For example, staff should not remove eyeglasses and dentures or place call buttons out of reach. The bed should be located next to the bathroom and the light left on to prevent falls. A patient should not be labeled "incontinent" when he or she has been restrained in bed and left unattended.
- Hospital-based case managers should encourage community-based case managers to follow their patients into the hospital and to orient acute

care staff about the patients' life-styles and functional levels before hospitalization. This will enable hospital staff to work to maintain, regain, or enhance prehospital functional levels. It is critically important that hospital staff understand the elderly patient's preadmission functional levels. A simple functional assessment will be enlightening in this regard.

- Hospitals should seek to actively support and bolster the informal care-giving network of churches, volunteers, friends, family, and neighbors, particularly in communities where cultural differences and nuances may require greater sensitivity. For example, hospitals could work through churches to accomplish the same ends with all elderly, regardless of cultural background.

- Hospitals could consider partnering with groups such as The National Association of Professional Geriatric Care Managers, in Tucson, to offer private care management services to those geriatric patients who need it and want to pay for it. In its role as a resource center, the hospital could also provide these services through a subcontracting arrangement.

- Hospitals, especially in rural areas, should strive to become service hubs that provide or sponsor community-based services such as adult day care, Meals-on-Wheels, congregate dining, nursing home services, assisted living, and other programs best suited to a safe campus setting. The hospital should become a comfortable community meeting place where the elderly can come for coffee and donuts, to play cards, or browse a lending resource library of videotapes and health care consumer pamphlets.

- If hospitals purchase and use mobile vans, the vans should be used for more productive purposes than blood pressure screening, ear wax removal, and other arguably wasteful uses of such a costly resource. Instead, vans might be used to perform functional assessments and to make house calls to homebound elderly who need physicals, mammograms, and dental care.

- Hospitals could develop respite care programs to give family caregivers a break. Such services, provided either in the hospital step-down or transitional care unit or at an affiliated nursing home, could be paid for out-of-pocket by the family.

• Innovative Hospital Programs for the Elderly

A number of hospitals nationwide are working to implement some of these ideas. St. Peter's Hospital (part of the Eastern Mercy Health System) in Albany, New York, provides a complete continuum of services for the elderly, with the acute care hospital at its hub. Services include a 160-bed nursing home, an adult day-care program, congregate living apartments, an assisted living facility, home care, rehabilitation, durable medical equipment, home infusion therapy, Meals-on-Wheels, Lifeline (emergency call) capacity, a community-based case management program, and an extensive volunteer program. Catherine McAuley Health System in Ann Arbor, Michigan, offers one-stop shopping for older adult services, including an Alzheimer's program and geriatric health services as well as community-based services for older adults. The system plans to expand its program by adding more physicians, nurses, and social workers specializing in the care of older adults and by providing a full range of education and support services to assist families in making informed decisions.

These early leaders in case management for the elderly demonstrate that everyone — acute and long-term care providers, older clients and their families, and health care and managed care social services — need to work together to "break down the walls, work more inclusively, and focus on prevention and wellness."[7]

• Conclusion

It is fair to ask, Who will pay for all of this? Many of these suggestions could be implemented at little or no cost, involving simply a shift in attitude, emphasis, or priority. Others might require a modest investment. And still others might require a substantial funding commitment. However, before sweeping change can occur, a nationwide public consensus must be developed to divert some of the funding away from high-tech, institution-based acute care toward relatively low-tech, community- and family-based services as well as to services that focus on prevention and wellness. Additionally, more creative and effective ways need to be developed to cultivate the present informal but effective care-giving system, which today provides 80 percent of all care for the elderly.[8-10]

Forward-looking hospitals can position themselves to coordinate and provide the services the elderly and their families really need and want. The future leaders in this field already are establishing case management programs characterized by a strong focus on community- and family-based care giving, sound functional assessments, and a growing sensitivity toward a culture that is rebuilding the very foundation of health and social services for its elders.

References

1. Amara, R. J., Morrison, J. D., and Schmid, G. *Looking Ahead at American Health Care.* Washington, DC: McGraw-Hill Book Co., 1988.

2. Kulczycki, M. T., ed. *The Hospital's Role in Caring for the Elderly: Leadership Issues.* Chicago: American Hospital Association (The Hospital Research & Educational Trust), 1982.

3. Persily, N. A., ed. *Eldercare: Positioning Your Hospital for the Future.* Chicago: American Hospital Publishing, 1991.

4. Taueber, C. M., and Goldstein, A. A. *Growth in America's Oldest Old Population. No. 2, Profiles of America's Elderly.* Washington, DC: Age & Sex Statistics Branch, Population Division, Bureau of Census, July 1992.

5. Amara, Morrison, and Schmid.

6. Taueber and Goldstein.

7. Miner, M. Personal communication, Senior Care Connection, Troy, NY, Nov. 9, 1992.

8. Amara, Morrison, and Schmid.

9. Family Service America. *The Family Guide to Elder Care: Making the Right Choices.* Milwaukee: FSA, 1990.

10. Persily.

Chapter 9

Case Management Model: Pediatrics

Linda Waite Maurano

• Introduction

The pediatric outpatient case management program must address several basic assumptions that are unique to the administration and supervision of pediatric care. Pediatric experts across the United States agree that pediatric care extends across a broad continuum involving many players. The successful pediatric case management model coordinates this continuum, recognizing that the transition from hospital to home is an ongoing process requiring constant evaluation and accommodation of changing status and case progression, while allowing for maximum utilization of available resources. Although pediatric case management programs may vary from hospital to hospital, one fundamental premise holds true: The *family*, not the patient, is the unit of care. Because families are an integral part of the care team and assume primary responsibility for their children's care, it is their strengths and weaknesses that are most critical to the success of the plan of care.

The goal of a comprehensive pediatric case management program is to provide appropriate services in a collaborative process that stresses education, problem solving, and advocacy and that supports the medically fragile child and the family alike by allocating every available resource to promote cost-effective, high-quality care. Through the painstaking but focused efforts of professionals from many disciplines, Children's National Medical Center in Washington, DC, has established a program that meets this ambitious goal. This chapter describes the evolution of the pediatric outpatient case management model implemented at Children's National Medical Center and explains the model's success.

• Basic Assumptions for Program Development

Several basic assumptions must be incorporated into the development of any pediatric case management program. These include:

- *Advances in research and medical technology have dramatically improved both the length and quality of life* for children who formerly might have had very short lives or required institutionalization.
- *Families are eager to learn care techniques* so that they can take their children home to a less restrictive environment and regain control over their lives with a sense of parental and familial competency.
- *Pediatric home care is unique,* so an agency that deals primarily with adult or elderly patients should not be the agency of choice to provide care for a medically fragile child whose health might decline rapidly and create a medical emergency.
- *All home care programs are not created equal,* and to be effective, a pediatric program must meet certain basic criteria.
- *Team members must collaborate* to provide effective, efficient care that will produce sound outcomes.
- *Case management is a core management tool* — an integral part of a high-quality, cost-effective health management system.

• Evolution of a Program Model

The pediatric case management model implemented at Children's National Medical Center evolved from previous attempts at facilitating the early hospital discharge of medically fragile children. Initial endeavors at case management used a team approach, involving the child's family, hospital staff, physicians, discharge planners, case managers employed by third-party payers, and home care staff. Unfortunately, because each discipline had its own agenda, efforts to bridge disciplines resulted in uncoordinated, dysfunctional, fragmented, and often duplicative care. Turf issues abounded. Each discipline had its own perception of the problem, and none seemed to appreciate the other's role in the overall process. Most intimidating of all, no one seemed to understand the uniqueness of pediatric patient care.

Families who felt they had effectively lost control over their lives wanted to take the hospitalized child home and attempt to regain a sense of normalcy. They wanted and needed to learn how to care for the child and to feel they were competent caregivers and parents, and they were frustrated at what they perceived to be a lack of empathy for their situation.

On the other hand, hospital staff and physicians worried about how the medically fragile child who had spent most of his or her life under *their* care in an intensive care setting could be safely discharged. Could the complex care they offered even be approximated in a nonhospital setting? When a child *was* discharged, their concerns were invariably confirmed by frequent calls from parents with complaints about the home care providers. These complaints included errors made by nurses who were accustomed to caring for adults, insufficient staffing, and the indiscriminate use of backup agencies.

Although discharge planners generally recognized the need for a discharge to the home, communicating with third-party payers' case managers about childrens' needs and suggested plans of care was often frustrating and time-consuming. Discharge planners felt that case managers chose home care programs based on cost alone, with no concern for their quality or for available resources — and without attention to feedback. It did not seem to matter that every referral of a medically complex child to certain home care programs appeared to end with an unplanned hospital readmission three to four days after discharge.

Payer-based case managers, in turn, expressed frustration with having to track down visiting staff to obtain current information on a child's condition, whereas the home care staff complained that they were kept so busy submitting verbal and written reports that the level of care they could offer the child suffered. In general, the home care staff did not seem to understand the need to communicate effectively with everyone else involved, especially with the insurance case managers, whose understanding and cooperation are essential to ensure continued approval of the home care plan.

Children's National Medical Center identified two primary barriers to the overall process: communication and education. Each discipline needed to recognize the benefits of integrated care and assigned accountability and to understand the intrinsic value of a focused and multidisciplined case management program. The Center was not alone in identifying such concerns. In two national think tanks assembled in 1992, composed of case managers and pediatric care providers from all over the nation, the predicaments were identical and without resolution. The think tanks were convened to lay the groundwork for development of an effective case management model of care especially designed for pediatric clients and their families. Specifically, the goals of the think tanks were to develop a pediatric case management model that would provide the following:

- A systematic approach to identifying high-risk and high-cost patients as early as possible
- A mechanism for coordinating the care of such patients
- Treatment planning to ensure quality by selecting care alternatives and providers best suited for the patient
- Total patient care management to achieve optimal outcomes

The think tanks generated a list of issues and realities to be incorporated in the pediatric case management philosophy. These included:

- Children's hospitals should coordinate inpatient and outpatient care, but most do not designate case managers to oversee inpatient care and expedite a smooth transition to the home care setting.
- Providers of pediatric services need access to case managers with pediatric experience. The case managers in attendance noted that 60 to 70 percent

of case managers *do* have pediatric experience and recommended that providers request a pediatric case manager specifically. If none was available, the hospital and the home care pediatric specialist would then have to explain in detail the specifics of the case, stressing the differences between pediatric and adult situations.

- Pediatric providers should assist case managers by requesting that case management be provided by the insurer/carrier. This should occur at the *onset* of hospitalization, not at discharge.
- Pediatric providers should help educate case managers by developing criteria for (1) the selection of home care providers based on quality and (2) the subsequent evaluation and monitoring of home-based services.
- Case managers need a mechanism to evaluate home care providers' *true* level of pediatric expertise.[1]

Another group of case managers representing a variety of insurers/carriers, ranging from health maintenance organizations (HMOs) to independents, held ongoing meetings in conjunction with Children's Home Health Care Services (CHHCS) in Washington, DC. Children's Home Health Care Services is a pediatric agency affiliated with Children's National Medical Center and provides the coordinated services of a home health agency, private-duty nursing agency, hospice, home medical equipment, and home infusion therapies. These meetings yielded results similar to those of the think tanks, except that the CHHCS group also stressed the need for forming partnerships in order to collaborate, communicate effectively, and coordinate the most appropriate care plan for the patient. The group acknowledged by consensus that care planning needs to be viewed as an ongoing process from hospital to home, able to accommodate the changing status and progress of the case, while allowing for the maximum use of all available resources.[2]

• Implementation and Success of the Program Model

The success of the Children's National Medical Center model is based on the assignment of case management responsibilities to a single professional for each patient. Thus, when the referral or discharge planning process begins in the inpatient or private sectors, the home care professional nurse becomes the case manager. This professional then becomes the focal point for all interventions, communication, and collaboration among hospital and home care staff, parents, allied health professionals, and third-party payer case managers. He or she also assumes the roles of negotiator, educator, and advocate, taking on responsibility for assessing needs, developing the plan, and facilitating its implementation in direct communication with all concerned. This person also is involved in clarifying roles and expectations and in evaluating options and available services.

The home care program offers distinct benefits to all concerned, particularly patients and families. The program provides the following:

- The least restrictive environment in which the child can grow and develop and the family can function as a unit
- Educational and support services that enable families to make the home an appropriate setting for delivering home health care services
- Assistance with identifying available community resources
- A coordinated home care plan that prevents duplication and fragmentation of services as well as undue family stress
- Peace of mind that the child is cared for by a pediatric specialist who is trained to detect when the child is becoming unstable and who will alert the health care team into action to prevent emergencies
- Twenty-four-hour-a-day, seven-day-a-week coverage, both in-service and through an on-call system
- Assistance with helping families define their present needs and effectively plan for changes and the future
- Assistance with helping families feel as if they are competent caretakers and encouragement to take on an advocacy role for their child

The program also offers significant benefits to insurance case managers. Among these benefits are that the program:

- Decreases the total cost of medical care and services.
- Prevents unplanned readmissions to the hospital.
- Decreases length of hospitalization.
- Decreases inappropriate use of the emergency department (ED).
- Decreases calls by family members to physicians and case managers.
- Improves patient/family compliance with the plan of treatment.
- Fosters the collaborative relationship among physicians, home care, family, and case managers, because the home care staff become the "eyes and ears" for the whole team. Their observations and interventions provide the basis for informed, appropriate decision making.
- Eases the transition from hospital to home and assists the insurance company in achieving client satisfaction in both the care rendered and the care managed.

However, care must be taken to choose the correct agency as well as to confirm the appropriateness of care for the child in the home setting.

• Selection of Appropriate Home Care Candidates and Agencies

Not every child or family is a candidate for medical and clinical care in the home. Some home environments may not be conducive to good health or may lack the physical space or resources to support the necessary equipment and care applications. Factors to consider include:

- The safety of the home environment
- The ability of primary caregivers and their willingness to participate in patient care
- The expectation that the child's condition can be safely treated at home
- The comparative benefit of home care versus care in another setting

Informed decision making always provides a safer outcome for the patient. Before making decisions regarding visit frequency or hours of care required, the following components must be weighed:

- The patient's condition
- Other diagnoses
- The patient's stability
- Number of readmissions
- Any prior rehabilitation period
- Family stress factors and support systems

In planning a pediatric home care model outside the confines of a pediatric facility, the choice of a home care agency is paramount to the safe delivery of care. Quality standards for home care delivery vary among agencies, and some do not employ staff experienced in working with high-risk children and special technologies. Figure 9-1 presents guidelines for profiling an agency and its procedures to assist case managers in determining which agencies are best suited to participate in the care of a child; figure 9-2 (p. 148) explains important differences between pediatric and adult home care; and figure 9-3 (p. 149) lists several distinguishing characteristics of successful pediatric home care agencies. Careful planning and choosing home care programs that can work well with hospital discharge planners and case managers will enhance the overall success of pediatric outpatient case management.

• Quality and Outcomes

The proof of a program's success can be measured by its outcomes. The Children's National Medical Center program has indeed fulfilled its promise, as shown by the following outcome criteria:

- Hospital length of stay decreased from 6.9 to 6.1 days.
- Referrals for home care increased from 8.8 percent of hospital discharges to 11 percent.
- High-tech referrals increased from 56 patients to 96.

Figure 9-1. Choosing a Pediatric Home Care Agency

Standards

1. Is the agency licensed by the state (or all the states) in which it delivers services?
2. Is the agency Medicare/Medicaid certified?
3. Is the agency accredited by one of the voluntary accrediting bodies?
   - Joint Commission on Accreditation of Healthcare Organizations
   - National League for Nursing
4. Have any complaints against the agency been filed with the state regulating agency?
5. Is the agency bonded? Does the agency bond its employees, or do the employees carry bonding for themselves?
6. Does the agency provide professional liability insurance, or does it require the staff carry their own?
7. How long has the agency been operating in the community?
8. Has the agency provided references from hospital personnel, physicians, social workers, and families who have used it?
9. Is there a patient bill of rights and responsibilities?
10. Is there a patient/family grievance system?
11. How does the agency deal with after-hours concerns of families, staff, professionals?
12. Is there a professional nurse on call 24 hours a day?
13. What is the background of the intake coordinator?
14. What is the bilingual availability?

Services

1. What services are provided by this agency?
   - Intermittent skilled nursing
   - Occupational therapist
   - Hourly skilled nursing
   - Speech therapist
   - Hospice
   - Medical social services
   - Home health aide
   - Home infusion
   - Companion/sitter services
   - Home medical equipment
   - Physical therapist
2. Does the agency provide a complete written list of its services?
3. Does the agency confer with the physician before providing services?
4. Does the agency coordinate with the physician, case manager, family, and staff regarding the plan of care, changes, and outcomes? How?
5. Is care available on weekends and after regular hours?
6. What procedures does the agency use in an emergency?
7. Are the agency staff trained in CPR?

(Continued on next page)

Figure 9-1.   (Continued)

Utilization

1. What is the average length of stay of patients serviced by the agency?

2. What is the average hours of service provided to patients who need hourly care?

3. How are patients' needs assessed and services adjusted accordingly?

4. What is the average number of visits *per week* to patients by the following disciplines?

   - Skilled nursing
   - Respiratory therapist
   - Physical therapist
   - Home health aides
   - Occupational therapist
   - Medical social services
   - Speech therapist

5. What percentage of the patients are:

   - Neonates (under 1 year)
   - Pediatrics (1 to 18 years)
   - Adults (18 to 64 years)
   - Adults (65 years +)

6. What percentage of the patients receive:

   - Two to three visits per week
   - More than one visit per day
   - One visit per week
   - Twenty-four-hour service

Agency Personnel

1. Are the people who will provide the care agency employees, or do they become the patient's/family's employees?

2. Who is liable for an injury or accident to a provider of care in the patient's home?

3. Who is liable if a provider of care causes injury to the patient?

4. Who is responsible if an item is broken by the provider of care in a patient's home?

5. What kind of education, training, and experience do the agency personnel have?

6. Have the agency personnel met state licensing requirements for their profession? If so, how is this verified?

7. Are references required of agency personnel before they are hired? If so, are they work references or personal?

8. Does the agency have a full range of personnel or does it subcontract for staff? If it subcontracts, how does it ensure the reliability and competence of these personnel?

9. Will the agency assign the same person to the case for the length of stay?

10. Does the agency check with the patient/family to determine whether the staff assigned are satisfactory?

Figure 9-1. (Continued)

11. What happens when a patient/family complains about a staff member? Is he or she replaced? How long does it take to effect the replacement?

12. Is supervision of personnel provided? If so, what kind of supervision is provided? How often does supervision occur? Does the supervisor make home visits while the employee is present?

13. Do staff have job descriptions?

14. How are staff oriented to their job descriptions?

15. How is the skill level of the staff determined?

16. Is there any training given prior to assignment to ensure that staff have up-to-date knowledge in a given area (for example, ventilators, IV therapy)?

17. Does the agency have requirements for in-service training? If so, how are they implemented?

18. Does the agency require home health aides to be certified?

19. How much training and experience are home health aides required to have?

20. How are home health aides supervised?

21. Does the agency facilitate an interdisciplinary team approach when more than one discipline is involved? How?

22. Are patients/families involved in the formulation and implementation of the plan of care? How?

23. How do staff give physicians and case managers feedback on the patient's progress?

24. What percentage of the staff have more than one year of pediatric experience?

RN _____%   PT _____%   LPN _____%

OT _____%   HHA _____%   MSW _____%

RT _____%

Financial

1. Does the agency accept assignment of benefits?

2. Does the agency bill the third-party payer directly, or does it require the family to pay privately and then submit receipts for reimbursement?

3. Does the agency provide bundled billing or coordinated billing?

4. Will the agency negotiate rates?

5. Does the agency bill weekly or monthly or either?

6. Is there a separate charge for supervision?

7. Will the agency furnish required clinical documentation to validate a bill?

Figure 9-2. Differences between Pediatric and Adult Home Care

Pediatric diagnoses are different.

A. Numerous diagnoses are congenital.

    1. Management of these diagnoses needs to go far beyond treating the physical. Attention must be given to the child's developmental stage and the family's coping ability and support system. These conditions continue over a lifetime, and unlike adults who are newly diagnosed, these children never know what it is to be disease-free.

    2. As children progress through the developmental tasks, they need to learn their activities of daily living (ADL) differently from their peers and without the benefit of being able to imitate their parents and siblings.

    3. Children are not relearning a previously acquired skill as adults would. For example, an adult who is blinded is relearning ADLs. A child who was born blind needs to learn ADLs in a different way and, therefore, his or her initial learning experience is more difficult.

    4. Examples of common congenital diseases include hemophilia, cystic fibrosis, kidney disease, juvenile diabetes, congenital heart disease, muscular dystrophy, cleft palate, sickle-cell disease, spina bifida. Other diseases common to children are asthma, leukemia, and apnea.

B. Some pediatric diagnoses may stem directly from dysfunctional parenting. These include child abuse, nonorganic failure to thrive, Munchausen syndrome, or PEST (poor eating, sleeping, and temper tantrums) syndrome.

    1. Attention must be given to the family as the unit of care.

    2. A child's ability to emotionally handle his or her condition, regardless of its cause, is affected by the associated stressful events he or she experiences.

Pediatric treatments are unique.

Pediatric patients are unique in terms of the types, frequency, amount, and durations of their treatments and related equipment and supplies. These children are very medically fragile, and the slightest error could cause a medical emergency. For example, administering 0.5 mg of digoxin rather than 0.1 mg of digoxin would be life-threatening.

Developmental levels vary.

A. Adults have stabilized in their developmental levels, but children are still evolving through the stages. For example, their need to develop autonomy and trust is compounded by their urgent need for normalized experiences—experiences that need to be achieved through a variety of opportunities outside their rooms. This need for autonomy is compounded by the need for dependency on their caretaker due to their physical condition.

B. Children's developmental levels also affect their ability to communicate any distress to the caretaker. How does a toddler indicate a pain's source and intensity? How does the caretaker know what comfort measures really work or when a medication has been effective? Some diseases afflicting children are accompanied by pain and discomfort beyond the appreciation of the normal adult. The child does not have the capability to express this the way an adult can.

The family, whatever its composition, is the pivotal point for home care of children.

Family is important in the care of adults, but the primary focus of adult health care is to assist and teach patients to increase their own level of independent functioning. In pediatric home care, the staff teach and assist the family or caregiver to deliver the appropriate care to the child. Identifying this caregiver and teaching and supporting the care at times is the greatest challenge.

Figure 9-3. Distinguishing Characteristics of Successful Pediatric Home Care Agencies

- *The staff at all levels* (registered nurse, licensed practical nurse, physical therapist, occupational therapist, respiratory therapist, speech therapist, social worker, and home health aide) *have neonatal/pediatric experience.* To ask a professional nurse whose caseload is 95 percent elderly clients to occasionally care for the medically fragile child is asking for trouble. Pediatric diagnoses, medications and doses, care needs, and treatments are very different. This is a major risk and liability factor.

- *Orientation and in-service training are geared toward the staff's ability to keep up with the changes in technology and miniaturized equipment.* These technologies are virtually the lifeblood that allows medically fragile children to live outside the controlled hospital setting. Thus, educational sessions also must deal with the staff's ever-changing role. Pediatric home care staff are not caring for or teaching an adult to take on self-care responsibility but are caring for children and teaching their families to be primary and competent caregivers. Staff are not there to take over the role of the parents but to enhance and augment the parents' ability to care for a sick child, who depends on them to make difficult choices about his or her welfare and management. This often is a difficult role for the staff, who have been taught to "do." The sometimes conflicting goal of pediatric home care is to promote family independence.

- *The staff's role revolves around patient and family advocacy.* Home care staff must take the lead in facilitating, encouraging, and permitting families to constantly reevaluate, negotiate, and search for good solutions under current circumstances of their daily life without feeling guilty. Once the parents' decisions are made, the staff must assist and support families in relating this to the medical and insurance communities. The staff also understand and encourage the development of backup plans so that families have options to fall back on.

- *In a family crisis* (for example, suddenly having to care for a medically fragile child at home) *social services intervene to help families cope and appropriately utilize community resources.*

- *Clinical policies and procedures are geared toward pediatric practice.* This also is extended to the supplies and equipment needed to provide care.

- *Discharge planning is thorough.* Not only does the child's plan of care need to be developed prior to discharge, but the mechanism by which it will be implemented and the environment in which it will unfold must be taken into account. In order for parents to be comfortable taking a medically fragile child home, they need to understand and be taught the means and the methods of care. The home environment needs to be set up ahead of time with the necessary equipment, appropriate electrical outlets, physical accessibility, and so on. This cannot all occur in 24 hours. The goal is to have a smooth transition from hospital to home, maintaining the continuum of care for the patient as well as support for the family. An improperly planned discharge soon betrays itself in overwhelmed, highly stressed parents and caregivers, unplanned readmissions to the hospital, or frequent visits to the ED. Discharge planning is as much a coping mechanism as it is an environmental readiness plan.

- There were zero unplanned readmissions to the hospital for case-managed patients.
- Family satisfaction, as reported via the family satisfaction survey completed at hospital discharge, rose from 4.05 (maximum total score of 5.0) to 4.12.
- There were no recorded delays of hospital discharge due to lack of home care resources, availability, and readiness.

Perhaps the most important outcome is patient and family satisfaction. Parents have frequently and repeatedly expressed satisfaction in playing an integral role in a plan that allowed them to regain control over their lives and to establish collaborative partnerships with a professional team for the care and benefit of their child. Additionally, the model has fortified the Center's risk management program, because the case management process assures patients and families that every possible resource has been tapped.

• Cost Implications

Implementing the case management model involved a staff of five full-time equivalents—three for the hospital and two for the home care unit—at an approximate total cost of $190,000. The Center perceives this cost as an essential investment in the long-term financial stability of the institution. Stronger relationships between hospital-based and payer-based case managers improved the quality of patient care through improved communication and education and, ultimately, resulted in a decrease in expensive patient days in the hospital and the more prudent use of an ideally supportive and cost-effective environment—the home.

• Conclusion

Children's National Medical Center's newly instituted and highly effective pediatric case management model has met its original goals. It has evolved from a dysfunctional nonsystem to become a highly successful collaborative process that stresses education, problem solving, and advocacy; provides the medically fragile child and his or her family with appropriate services; and allocates available resources to promote cost-effective, high-quality care. Its successful maturation is the direct result of multidisciplined efforts of professionals focused on enhancing the management of pediatric outpatients and their families. Developing a high-quality, fully integrated pediatric case management program certainly posed its fair share of challenges. But the benefits to patients, their families, the hospital, and payers has been well worth the effort for the sake of this country's most valuable national resource—its children.

References

1. Child Health Corporation of America. *Pediatric Case Management: A National Think Tank.* Kansas City, MO: CHCA, 1992.

2. Children's Home Health Care Services. Pediatric Case Management Forum. Washington, DC: CHHCS, Dec. 1992.

Bibliography

Feinberg, E. A. Family stress in pediatric home care. *Caring* 7(5):38, May 1985.

Hamilton, B., and Vessey, J. Pediatric discharge planning. *Pediatric Nursing* 18(5):475, Sept.–Oct. 1992.

Klug, R. M. Selecting a home care agency. *Pediatric Nursing* 18(5):504, Sept.–Oct., 1992.

Maurano, L. W. Pediatric home care: past, present, and future. *Journal of Home Health Care Practice* 1(a):1–7, 1989.

Perrin, J. M. Chronically ill children in America. *Caring* 7(5):16, May 1985.

Chapter 10

Case Management Model: Emergency Department

Gail P. Loadman and Samuel J. Kiehl III, MD

• Introduction

Emergency departments (EDs), the leading providers of unscheduled primary and acute care in the country, are struggling to provide cost-effective treatment and safe disposition to appropriate levels of care. The local ED has become the primary health care resource for those whom society has failed to serve with other health care alternatives. But the contemporary emergency facility, though it offers a broad spectrum of care in a setting surrounded by an armamentarium of resources, is an ill-equipped medical provider of last resort for episodic and chronic illnesses. Patients are often ill-served and the specialized resources of EDs are inefficiently utilized in such situations.

This milieu presents an opportunity for several outpatient case management models that employ an interdisciplinary approach to assessment, intervention, and referral to more appropriate clinical settings. This chapter describes two case management models for emergency care: a payer model and a clinical model. Both models are designed to provide a continuum of care, quality controls, and effective cost containment for a diverse patient base with varied medical and social needs.

• The Payer Model

The payer case management (extraorganizational) model is built on a partnership between health maintenance organizations (HMOs) and emergency departments that teams HMO-based nurses and ED-based physicians as case managers. The HMO nurses answer members' phone calls and direct emergency cases to the triage officer of the day, a designated ED physician, for further clinical assessment and treatment or referral. This case management model has been implemented successfully at many hospitals despite significant barriers and disincentives among managed care organizations.

ED versus HMO Emergency Care

Although they play a principal role in improving access, enhancing quality, and reducing costs, hospital EDs often find themselves at odds with HMOs. As currently organized, the high cost of delivering acute and primary care in the ED has prompted many HMOs to create disincentives against ED visits. Still, these disincentives have not significantly deterred HMO enrollees from utilizing EDs across the country for all sorts of minor acute complaints requiring time-consuming preauthorization calls and, all too often, nonpayment for services provided.

Unfortunately, many managed care organizations have failed to offer hands-on alternative care options for after-hours care within their service areas. Although some HMOs provide 24-hour services (including urgent care), others offer limited office hours in conjunction with a "gatekeeper" call system that is often handled by a registered nurse. The gatekeeper system requires the ED to pursue a cumbersome preauthorization process for emergency workup, usually followed by repeated calls for admission or transfer of the patient to a participating hospital. There are documented downsides for the HMO as well as for the patient. For the HMO, these include high overhead and capital equipment costs, inefficiencies in patient scheduling, and space and staffing concerns to accommodate unscheduled acute illness with its accompanying fluctuating patient volumes. For patients, the primary dissatisfiers include treatment delays and additional out-of-pocket costs for nonauthorized visits.

Advantages of ED–HMO Partnerships

A partnering agreement between the ED and an HMO promotes the ED as a magnet center for managing unscheduled pediatric and adult acute care needs. A designated ED to provide after-hours pediatric, acute, and subacute care offers the HMO significant direct and indirect savings in overhead, staffing, and other costs, especially in communities with few alternatives for after-hours health care. The ED, of course, gains a rich source of referrals.

In forging a contractual agreement, the HMO and ED together establish standards of quality and practice parameters for specific presenting complaints. Capitated payment or cost-based per-encounter fees, practice guidelines, measures to ensure patient convenience and satisfaction, and referral mechanisms are all components of contract negotiation.

Many advantages have materialized from ED–HMO service delivery and case management partnerships. Patient dissatisfaction and poor outcomes as a result of shoddy phone triage are virtually eliminated. Medical management of the patient is prompt and promotes early diagnosis and treatment intervention with less risk of maloccurrence, progressive illness, and unnecessarily intense and extensive resource utilization. The medical care continuum is maintained by enhanced communication, documentation, and information networking between the HMO primary care providers and the ED physician.

The Role of Practice Guidelines

All future case management initiatives in the emergency department will include practice guidelines. Numerous state health reform proposals call for the use of practice guidelines to enhance patient management by addressing quality, cost, utilization, and professional liability. Emergency medicine provides a perfect opportunity to establish parameters for treating the most commonly presented injuries and illnesses, guiding physicians and patients toward the most highly productive and cost-effective diagnostic and therapeutic modalities.

Emergency diagnostic and therapeutic modalities today are largely driven by tradition or the practice of defensive medicine. Practice guidelines developed and accepted by emergency physicians can minimize (not eliminate) bad outcomes while eliminating many interventions of minimal incremental value. Such guidelines have been used successfully in some states to limit physician and hospital liability, to reduce underwriting costs, and to cap court awards for malpractice. By combining practice parameters with liability reform and medical review, government and commercial payers can lessen the burdens of patient micromanagement, ensure clinical quality, and get more value for every health care expenditure without selective rationing.

The following two examples illustrate the prudent application of practice guidelines in emergency care:

- A patient presents with nausea and vomiting. Though diagnostic testing might commonly include complete blood count (CBC), electrolytes, and an acute abdominal series. The value of all three of these tests is widely disputed, especially in cases where obstruction, gastrointestinal bleeding, or underlying chronic illnesses are unlikely. Establishing institutional guidelines that clarify when such tests would be useful and when they are of little use could save millions of dollars each year.
- A head-injured patient has experienced a brief loss of consciousness. Many physicians would obtain skull X rays and computed tomography (CT) scans followed by hospital admission for inpatient observation. But there are strong arguments against such a course of treatment: Skull X rays are necessary only when a penetrating injury is suspected; CT scans should be used sparingly; and, instead of a costly inpatient admission, a briefer stay in an observation unit may suffice to determine the need for further diagnostic or therapeutic intervention.

As the primary medical case manager, the emergency physician plays a crucial role in developing, following, and enforcing meaningful practice guidelines that reduce unnecessary and duplicative services while maintaining the quality of emergency care. Useful addendums to physician practice guidelines in the ED may include educational brochures describing common pathophysiological entities and diagnostic and treatment modalities to assist patients in understanding their disease process and the treatment rendered in the ED.

A Payer Model Case Study

A 20-year-old man, out joyriding on his motorcycle without a helmet, skids on some loose gravel and rolls his bike, sustaining many abrasions and a knot on his head. It is 11 o'clock at night and, as required by his health insurance carrier, the man phones the nurse on duty at his HMO, who gets a history over the phone and then calls the physician triage officer of the day. The triage physician has three choices:

1. He or she can get up and meet the patient at the office or the ED, taking time to dress, travel, wait for diagnostic results, and return home to an interrupted night's sleep.
2. He or she can redirect the patient to the office the following day, risking a conflict with scheduled appointments and, should the man suffer an overnight complication (such as subdural hematoma), likely allegations of inappropriate standards of care and medical negligence.
3. He or she can send the patient to an ED, where an alert, competent staff is available to examine the man and intervene as required.

The last choice seems the obvious one, even though it may cost more up front. Case management guidelines for the HMO nurse and the ED triage officer must incorporate proper incentives to direct patients to the most clinically appropriate and truly cost-effective resource—in this case, the emergency department.

• The Clinical Model

The majority of emergency departments employ a clinical (intradepartmental) model of case management that focuses on medical diagnosis and short-term clinical management, with due regard for social and aftercare needs. Emergency physicians and nursing professionals offer case management in a team approach enhanced by an integrated practice concept that combines high-level communication, practice protocols, and enhanced standards of care. The model has three chief components: diagnosis and therapy, observation services, and discharge planning and aftercare.

Diagnosis and Therapy

Over the past five years, payers and providers have embraced advancing diagnostic and therapeutic technologies to broaden the scope of hospital emergency services. Earlier diagnosis, more definitive and effective treatment, expanded observation capabilities, and thoughtful discharge planning have minimized ED morbidity, prevented inappropriate acute care admissions, and limited employer/employee lost work time due to illness. In contrast to office-based practices and freestanding urgent care facilities, which have limited on-site resources to handle serious trauma and medical illness, the hospital ED has immediate access to full laboratory services, X-ray and more sophisticated imagers, and the latest resuscitation equipment. In short, the ED is the most practical alternative for the diagnosis and treatment of unexpected acute illnesses and injuries. In the clinical model, the expert guidance of emergency physicians and nurses as case managers ensures that every client enjoys the full benefit of the ED's superior diagnostic and therapeutic resources.

Observation Services

The observation unit is the heart of the clinical model of emergency case management. By observing difficult-to-diagnose clients for a prolonged period, but without having to admit them to a hospital bed, physician and nurse case managers can take extra care and time in establishing the right diagnosis and recommending a proper course of treatment with utmost confidence.

In 1990, the American College of Emergency Physicians established a section for observational medicine. At that time, many EDs were already providing observation services informally in an effort to manage care more efficiently. Several forces have nurtured the advancement of observation services:

- The high cost of hospitalization and the ever-watchful, retrospective scope of peer review systems encouraged physicians to avoid inappropriate hospitalizations. A resultant increase in the incidence of bad outcomes spawned malpractice claims and skyrocketing malpractice insurance premiums. The pendulum then swung back, as physicians ordered more and more short-stay hospitalizations without documented findings.
- EDs often served as holding areas for critically ill patients when hospital critical care beds were full. Many critical care beds were taken up by patients experiencing chest pain who had been admitted to rule out myocardial infarction. Nationwide studies illustrated that fewer than 20 percent of these patients had actually suffered an acute myocardial infarction (AMI). A better methodology for diagnosing and housing chest pain patients was needed to treat those who lacked EKG or other significant

evidence of AMI without jeopardizing the 4 to 5 percent who genuinely were at risk.

- Many patients were too sick or posed too great a risk for safe discharge but failed to meet the criteria required for acute care hospital admission. Elderly patients especially often fell into this subacute category and required a short-stay alternative for intermediate or definitive care.
- Analyses of short-stay hospitalizations revealed frequent inefficient and excessively long stays due to poor management of the diagnostic and therapeutic regime in the hospital. Without a physician readily available and a well-designed care management plan to expedite patient care through a number of decision points, hospital days are wasted, illnesses are prolonged, lengths of stay are extended, hospital beds become scarce, and hospital costs routinely exceed diagnosis-related group (DRG) reimbursement.

Observational medicine blossomed to fill these voids. Staffed by emergency nurses and physicians, the observation unit provides safe, efficient, and high-quality clinical case management for a variety of patient types.

The observation unit at Riverside Methodist Hospital in Columbus, Ohio, provides an example of the benefit of observation services in the case-managed era. In 1988, Dr. John Picken, director of quality enhancement, studied a group of patients diagnosed with chest pain of undetermined cause who were admitted to monitored hospital beds. He discovered that approximately 15 percent of these patients had acute myocardial infarction. He further noted that the average length of stay (ALOS) for the 85 percent who had not suffered an AMI exceeded three days.

The following year, an observation unit was established with six monitored beds hard-wired to a central nursing station monitor. Patients at low risk for AMI were admitted to this unit when they had chest pain of undetermined cause. Statistical analysis of this group was similar to Dr. Picken's findings in that 15 percent turned out to have myocardial problems and required hospitalization. However, the other 85 percent were candidates for discharge. This process of case management on the observation unit required an average of 14 hours. The observation unit thus saved innumerable admissions, made critical care beds more available for critically ill patients, enhanced patient flow into Riverside's critical care unit from outlying referring hospitals, allowed hospital admissions from the ED to flow much more smoothly, and curtailed the diversion of emergency squads from Riverside's ED.

A number of diagnoses may warrant admission to the observation unit. Table 10-1 lists the 10 most common diagnoses for observation unit patients at Riverside Hospital; the average lengths of stay for these conditions are noted in table 10-2. Figure 10-1 illustrates the growing utilization of observation services at Riverside. As payers insist on safer and more cost-effective emergency care, the short-stay observation unit will become an attractive high-quality alternative in the case management continuum.

Discharge Planning and Aftercare

Most hospital ED patients are discharged home following diagnosis and initial treatment, creating a potentially gaping hole in the care continuum. The appropriate management of follow-up care for emergency patients is fundamental to an effective case management process. As the population ages and ED volumes escalate, aftercare management will become more comprehensive and complex than ever. Ensuring safe discharge in contemporary

Table 10-1. Percentage of Patients Admitted and Discharged after Observation, by Diagnosis

Diagnosis	Total Number of Patients	Percentage of Patients Admitted	Percentage of Patients Discharged
1. Chest pain	2,115	25.4	74.6
2. Abdominal pain	655	25.6	74.4
3. Respiratory disorders	633	36.8	63.2
4. Urologic disorders	470	33.1	66.9
5. Neurologic disorders	460	35.6	64.4
6. Dysrhythmia	444	36.9	63.1
7. Syncope	243	33.7	66.3
8. CHF	187	59.8	40.2
9. Pain syndromes	169	28.9	71.1
10. Vomiting	165	23.6	76.4

Table 10-2. Average Length of Stay in the Observation Unit

Diagnosis	Percentage Admitted to Hospital	ALOS in the Observation Unit (hours)	LOS in Observation Unit (hours), Discharged Patients
1. Chest pain	8.09	12.64	14.29
2. Abdominal pain	9.26	10.46	10.90
3. Respiratory disorders	8.03	11.20	13.10
4. Urologic disorders	8.91	12.02	13.60
5. Neurologic disorders	6.78	9.98	11.75
6. Dysrhythmia	7.29	11.25	13.58
7. Syncope	7.03	11.40	13.58
8. CHF	7.09	9.14	12.31
9. Pain syndromes	10.32	11.71	12.27
10. Vomiting	9.04	11.84	12.69

Figure 10-1. Utilization of Observation Services at Riverside

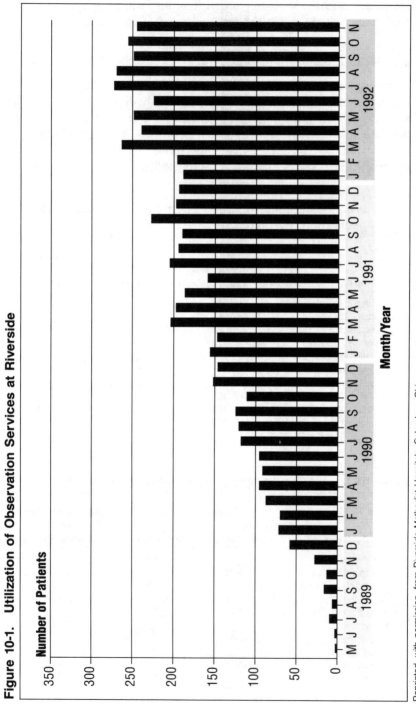

practice involves the management of medical, clinical, and social needs—including transportation and access to pharmaceuticals, durable medical equipment, home care, and, more and more frequently, shelter. Traditionally, such aftercare services were coordinated by nursing and physician staff, but the overburdened staff in today's crowded EDs are ill-equipped to handle the growing number of clients with complex social problems. For high-volume EDs, especially in urban hospitals, an outpatient case manager dedicated to emergency aftercare is an invaluable resource.[1]

According to Dr. Laurence Gavin, a well-planned discharge from the ED has six distinguishing characteristics. These are:[2]

1. Careful consideration of the psychosocial, financial, and medical factors that affect patient care
2. Appropriate aftercare treatment and follow-up arrangements
3. Effective education of the patient and any significant others
4. Safe transportation to a suitable living environment
5. Critical review of discharge plans and outcomes as part of a comprehensive quality assurance program
6. Satisfactory compliance with relevant laws, regulations, policies, and risk management principles

An Aftercare Case Study

An elderly female, Mrs. H, arrives by squad in the ED. She fell at home, having slipped on an area rug, and presents with pain and tenderness in the left ankle and right shoulder. Following examination and interpretation of her X rays, it is determined that she has sustained an ankle sprain and a bruised right shoulder. A double schanz wrap is applied to the left ankle.

Usual home care instructions following these relatively minor injuries might include: application of ice to the injured areas during the next 24 to 48 hours; use of crutches for one week or until pain-free; and follow-up with an orthopedic specialist as needed. A prescription for medication for pain relief would be provided.

The nurse case manager and a social worker collaboratively perform an individualized assessment and identify the following factors in planning Mrs. H's discharge:

- Mrs. H lives alone in a second-floor apartment. She has lived in the apartment for three months, having moved there from her family home of 40 years. Many of her new neighbors also are elderly. Discussion of this significant life change evokes an emotional, tearful response.
- She has one son who lives within 30 minutes of the hospital. He is recuperating from surgery performed one week ago.
- Transportation to return home cannot be identified by Mrs. H.

- Use of crutches will not be appropriate due to the shoulder injury and her normal unsteady gait.
- Activities of daily living, such as toileting, bathing, and meal preparation, will be difficult to impossible.
- Mrs. H will not be able to make the trip to her local pharmacy to obtain the prescription for pain medication.

An aging population, changing family structures, and the need for skilled care combine to create similar scenarios in the ED every day. Obviously, compliance with the usual discharge home would be low. A holistic, comprehensive approach to aftercare for Mrs. H is clearly indicated.

To meet Mrs. H's complex needs, the social worker or case manager contacts a variety of community and hospital resources, family, and friends. An assessment of her financial resources must precede intervention. Facilitating a comprehensive approach to aftercare may require EDs to develop and maintain on-site pharmaceutical and medical supplies as well as other direct services, which could be incorporated in a global bill. Patients often do not have money to purchase needed equipment and pharmaceuticals at the time of discharge from an ED, or it may be difficult to find pharmacies and equipment dealers that are conveniently located, open, and properly stocked.

A number of discharge outcomes were effected for Mrs. H. They included the following:

- Her care was managed in the ED observation unit for 6 hours.
- Ice was applied to the injured areas; a meal was provided; and pain medication was provided, which caused drowsiness and nausea.
- A different medication was prescribed and the prescription obtained from the in-house pharmacy prior to discharge.
- A walker for home use was accessed via the medical supply room. The physical therapist spent 30 minutes, just prior to discharge, instructing and demonstrating how to use the walker.
- A home health service will provide assistance with activities of daily living twice each day for five to seven days. Discussion with the service included the need for an environmental assessment, particularly the need to remove the area rug that caused Mrs. H's fall.
- Mrs. H's primary care physician was contacted. He made a referral to an orthopedist. An appointment was made prior to discharge. A copy of the ED record was forwarded to both the primary care physician and the orthopedist.
- A friend from the "old neighborhood" provided transportation home.

• Conclusion

The emergency department surely will play a pivotal role in health care reform efforts and restructured delivery systems. Organized case management philosophies and paradigms are fundamental to addressing the hottest reform topics: quality, utilization, cost, and professional liability. The new reality will present many emergency care alternatives, including the strategic flexibility to provide several outpatient case management models.

Extraorganizational (the payer model) and intradepartmental (the clinical model) partnerships hold great promise for restructuring emergency care delivery systems, improving the quality of care, and saving untold health care dollars. But such promises will soon be broken without an organized system that provides a continuum of high-quality care for the growing number of patients who will require case management services within or beyond the scope of the ED.

Outpatient case management is critical to the future provision of emergency care and must be considered an investment that will meet community health and social needs while improving the fiscal well-being of payers and providers alike.

References

1. Donovan, M. R. An endangered resource. *Health Progress* 72(4):50–54, May 1991.

2. Gavin, L. J. Discharge planning. In: R. A. Hellstern, editor. *Managing the Emergency Department: A Team Approach.* Dallas: American College of Emergency Physicians, 1992.

Chapter 11 _____

Case Management Model: Hospice

Judith A. Lebanowski

• Introduction

In the nearly two decades since the hospice concept was initiated in the United States, the movement has grown from an alternative health care choice to an integrated part of the country's health care system, with more than 1,800 hospice programs nationwide. The creation of a hospice Medicare benefit as part of the Tax Equity and Fiscal Responsibility Act of 1982 contributed to this growth by recognizing hospices as distinct providers offering medically appropriate care and the significant potential for cost savings.

The hospice care program at Riverside Methodist Hospital in Columbus, Ohio, is an excellent example of provider-based outpatient case management that consistently achieves positive outcomes for clients, payers, and the community. This chapter discusses the hospice concept from implementation of the program to the financial incentives it offers the hospital, and examines in particular the Riverside model.

• The Hospice Concept

Hospice is an example of provider-based case management. It is both a philosophy of care and a coordinated network of medical and supportive services designed to optimize quality of life for terminally ill patients and their families. Hospice program design is based on the following basic tenets:

- Hospice care focuses on enhancing quality of life and providing a comfortable, dignified death.
- Effective pain and symptom management is primary.
- Care is delivered by an interdisciplinary team of physicians, nurses, social workers, counselors, therapists, home hospice aides, pharmacists, dietitians, clergy, and extensively trained volunteers.

- The hospice treats the needs of the whole patient—physical, emotional, social, and spiritual—and the whole family system.
- Patient choices are honored.
- Care in the home is encouraged.
- Services are available 24 hours a day, 7 days a week.
- Death is seen as a natural part of the life progression and thus is neither hastened nor postponed.
- Bereavement care continues for the family for up to one year.

Hospice programs serve persons of all ages who have a terminal diagnosis with a prognosis of six months or less. Nationally, 84 percent of hospice patients have a diagnosis of cancer; other diagnoses include end-stage heart, lung, kidney, and neurological disease and AIDS.[1] Generally, care is provided regardless of ability to pay.

• Program Implementation

Successful implementation of a hospice program of care begins with a visioning and strategic planning process that includes a broad constituency. Several key areas should be addressed in implementing a hospice program.

The need for a new program should be assessed and existing community resources for the terminally ill evaluated. If other hospice programs exist, what percentage of the terminally ill are being served? Are existing services reaching persons of color, children, persons with diagnoses other than cancer, the poor, persons living alone or in nursing facilities?

The scope of services and where and how they will be provided should be defined. A comprehensive continuum of hospice care would include information and referral, home care, inpatient care (for both symptom management and respite), day care, residential care (for patients without a family caregiver), bereavement care, and community education. Generally, inpatient care is provided through arrangements with hospitals or skilled nursing facilities, but many are choosing to build hospice care centers that offer the advantages of a peaceful, homelike setting free from technology and dedicated to caring for the dying. At a minimum, the hospice must meet federal hospice Medicare regulations as well as state licensure and Medicaid regulations, if applicable.

High-quality leadership should be selected. The hospice executive director and medical director must be committed to the hospice philosophy and must become knowledgeable regarding hospice mission, services, staffing, reimbursement, and regulations.

The hospice organizational structure and governance should be considered. All aspects of the hospice program must be centrally administered, combining a high degree of autonomy with clear accountability for outcomes.

Networking should be undertaken. Possible avenues for networking include the National Hospice Organization, the state organization, and other hospice providers in the region.

• Barriers to Implementation

Barriers to successful implementation can be both external and internal. The hospice concept is an anomaly in our largely death-denying society, and admission to a hospice program often is seen as giving up or taking away hope. Widespread education is the appropriate long-term strategy to overcome this barrier. Hospice administrators and practitioners should be actively involved in educational programs at medical and nursing schools and in the community at large.

Hospice Medicare regulations requiring a six-month or less prognosis may create a barrier for physicians reluctant to certify a patient's life expectancy. To overcome this barrier, hospice professionals themselves are developing greater expertise in prognostication.

Internally, restrictive admission criteria and policies — for example, requiring a 24-hour caregiver in the home or admitting only do-not-resuscitate (DNR) patients — might wrongly exclude patients and families who are struggling to come to terms with a terminal diagnosis. Program administrators should be careful not to interpret hospice philosophy or Medicare regulations too rigidly.

Finally, it must be recognized that hospices have served a largely middle class, white, educated population. The hospice model of care must continue to evolve, and its reimbursement mechanisms must be redesigned to provide equal access to all persons, while continuing to ensure quality.

• Financial Incentives for Hospice Programs

There are clear financial incentives for a hospital considering implementation of a hospice program. The hospice model of outpatient case management supports the desirable shift from acute inpatient services to community-centered outpatient or ambulatory care services with an emphasis on maintaining the well-being of both patient and family in the midst of loss. With 24-hour on-call response and a focus on proactive interventions and family teaching, home-based hospice care significantly reduces acute inpatient days and emergency department visits and, so, reduces the Medicare diagnosis-related group (DRG) losses suffered when terminally ill patients are admitted to the acute care setting. Integrated systems of hospitals and hospices working together, formally or informally, allow the more timely identification and transfer of hospice-appropriate patients to hospice home care or to the hospice inpatient or residential care setting. In addition, bereavement care for the family helps reduce symptoms and illness associated with unresolved grief and loss. In short, as an outpatient model of case management, the hospice helps reduce overall health care costs.

Several studies have demonstrated that substantial cost savings are possible when hospice care replaces traditional acute hospital care for the terminally ill person in the last year of life.[2] Statistics gathered from Medicare-certified hospice programs since 1983 show that 90 to 95 percent of all hospice patient days occur in the home rather than in conventional health care settings.[3] Early referrals to hospice result in the greatest cost benefits by allowing "hospice-managed care" to appreciably replace other high-cost alternatives during the last months of life.

• Communication and Commitment for a Continuum of Care

The effective medical management of hospice patients hinges on communication both with physicians and among hospice team members. First, the hospice interdisciplinary team — physicians, nurses, social workers, counselors, therapists, home hospice aides, pharmacists, dietitians, clergy, and extensively trained volunteers — must establish positive partnerships with referring physicians, enabling them to see hospice as an extension of their practices. Medical school and continuing education does little to prepare physicians for dealing with quality of life issues in terminal illness. Many are uncomfortable when dealing with the dying patient and his or her family. When the hospice positions itself in partnership with the physician, it becomes easier for the physician to shift the focus of care to comfort and quality, assuring the patient and family that he or she will continue to support them through the hospice team.

• The Riverside Model

Hospice at Riverside provides a continuum of family-centered care to meet the individualized needs of both patient and family, including information and referral, home care, day care, inpatient care (both for symptom management and respite), residential care (for patients without a family caregiver), bereavement care, and community education. *Family* is defined as anyone who shares the patient's life and is important to his or her well-being, including friends, significant others, and pets. This approach requires a broad interdisciplinary team, which includes massage therapists, more than 200 specially trained volunteers, and a hospice "canine companion" who lives at Hospice at Riverside.

Hospice services are provided out of a freestanding facility, which houses the day care program, home care teams, and the administrative offices. Palliative inpatient care is provided in a nine-bed unit with a homelike atmosphere, complete with pet therapy and devoid of threatening technology or uniformed staff. Its genuine residential ambience is comfortable for both patient and family.

Medical and psychosocial care management begins with an initial referral and program admissions process. Once referred, the initial assessment of patient and family is performed by a registered nurse, who determines the need for either acute hospice or outpatient home care services. Level-of-care requirements and site-of-care determinations are dependent on this primary assessment, as are case management assignments and accountability. Following this assessment, the hospice interdisciplinary team (including the patient's attending physician) develops a comprehensive plan of care reflecting the patient's/ family's priorities and assigns a *family case manager*—a registered nurse whose ultimate responsibility lies in coordinating the entire continuum of services. Each family also is assigned a social worker and generally a home hospice aide, and a volunteer. Other team services, including chaplain, psychologist, massage therapist, and dietitian, are referred as needed. As these patients may alternate between home and inpatient care services, this infrastructure contributes to an organized team approach essential for promoting a seamless continuum of care.

Clear, open communication among the hospice interdisciplinary team members is critical to effective medical management and appropriate levels-of-care administration. The team meets formally every week to plan, review, and evaluate the plan of care for each patient. In more informal daily meetings, considerable attention is paid to communication among team members, on-call staff, and inpatient staff. This kind of communication ensures a holistic approach to care and provides continuity for the patient and family.

To create and sustain this kind of work environment, the team members' own personal needs must be taken into account. The organizational structure must reflect a collaborative approach, and hospice administrators must be strongly committed to staff support and renewal and must recognize the impact on the staff of chronic grief and loss. Cross-training of home care and inpatient staff, flexible scheduling, and "mental health" days are helpful ways to support staff renewal.

• Quality and Cost Monitors

Monitoring quality and cost are essential functions of a hospice program. Because the foundation of hospice is the alleviation of pain and suffering, the effectiveness of total pain management must be monitored, and pain must be approached from a holistic perspective. Ideally, data should be collected from patient or family interviews as well as from the clinical record.

Hospice administrators must help the entire organization make a meaningful connection between quality management activities and the hospice mission. An effective quality management program will give boards and staffs the confidence to expand services and achieve high productivity while maintaining consistently high quality services.

By establishing a statistical and financial data base and clearly defining categories and levels of care, costs can be allocated appropriately to determine the cost per patient day. Development of a cost accounting framework that reflects the cost of doing business will allow the hospice to track actual costs per day, set appropriate charges, and demonstrate the value of hospice care to payers. Per diem risk-based reimbursement generally is the benefit of choice for hospice case-managed care.

• Market-Conscious Strategies

Marketing strategies for hospice must focus on the key customers who participate in making the hospice care decision. These include:

- The patient
- The family or caregiver
- The attending physician
- The medical care system, including the payer
- The hospice program admissions staff

Each customer has different expectations, and a decision to enter the hospice program will not occur until all are in alignment. Because the physician is the key influencer in referring patients and families to hospice, marketing strategies should focus on that key customer. The hospice must view physicians as its primary customers, learn what their needs are, and develop a plan to meet those needs.

Of course, the effective marketing strategy will focus on building relationships with all customers, including the payers. Marketing strategies also must address internal hospice operations, including response time from referral to admission, admission criteria, patient-sensitive policies, and consistent communication with the attending physician throughout the course of hospice care. Lastly, well-informed, involved staff and volunteers who feel ownership of the hospice organization and mission will contribute significantly to the program's overall marketing effort.

• Conclusion

The hospice movement is transforming the dying process in the United States just as Lamaze transformed the birthing process. In many ways, the very presence of a hospice program enhances the quality of life of the entire community. Because it has evolved as a quality service industry that emphasizes compassion, the hospice movement has enjoyed the support of legislators, payers, and consumers alike.

Continued success of the hospice concept will depend in large part on a continued commitment to the hospice mission as the industry grows to serve new populations and new communities. The Riverside model offers a paradigm of hospice case management that provides high-quality, cost-effective, and holistic care to patients with a limited life expectancy and their families.

References

1. 1990 Census Data. Arlington, VA: National Hospice Organization.

2. Moga, D. W. The hospice equation. *Business and Health,* June 1985, pp. 7–11.

3. Hospice Organization of Wisconsin. *Hospice Guidelines for Establishing a Hospice Benefit in a Health Care Plan.* Madison, WI: Hospice Organization of Wisconsin, 1990.

Chapter 12

Case Management Model: Rural Home Care

Cherie Weber

• Introduction

Home care case management in the rural setting is indisputably challenging for patients, providers, practitioners, and payers. Health care delivery in vast, sparsely populated areas has always met with an array of barriers foreign to other geographic regions. Today, with more than 25 percent of the nation's population residing in rural America, enhancing the access to care for these medically underserved citizens is a chief concern.

Providing home care in rural areas holds great promise, but successful implementation ultimately hinges on the availability of practitioners, support staff, and regional resources. Properly conceived, implemented, and operated hospital-based home care programs are an excellent way to provide home care services and to make accessible the full range of health care resources to homebound individuals across many country miles.

Having overcome some of the seemingly insurmountable barriers to providing rural home care, the case management model established at Illinois Valley Community Hospital home care department is successfully serving the home care needs of Peru, Illinois, and its surrounding rural communities. This chapter discusses the many types of barriers to providing rural home care services and, using the experiences of Illinois Valley Community Hospital, describes how those barriers may be overcome.

• Barriers to Rural Case Management

The barriers to providing home care in rural areas may be divided into four broad categories. These are:

1. Philosophical and operational differences among hospital, home care, and outpatient policies and procedures, both clinical and administrative

2. A limited supply of appropriate and qualified home care staff
3. A geographically large service area, posing certain difficulties in access, communication, and transportation
4. A limited supply of ancillary and support services and resources

Philosophical and Operational Barriers

Decades of exclusively providing inpatient care have left hospitals with organizational, management, resource, and clinical policies focused on the patient lying in a hospital bed. Long dependent on inpatient revenues for fiscal survival, many hospitals found it nearly impossible to follow the rapid shift toward home care delivery following implementation of Medicare's prospective payment system.

For small rural facilities especially, a deeply embedded inpatient care culture and declining reimbursement rates over the past decade precluded development of home care services. But some facilities managed to establish new visions and missions and, guided by new values and philosophies, created innovative and integrated home care delivery systems — hospital-based home health care agencies.

Staffing Barriers

Regardless of size or organizational structure, rural home care agencies require a full complement of appropriately skilled staff to provide in-home services. Registered nurses, certified nurses' aides, medical social workers, and physical, occupational, and speech therapists are in increasing demand in rural areas, especially for home care services.

A Medicare-certified hospital-based home care department further requires qualified administrative, supervisory, and clerical staff. Recruitment of competent office staff is fundamental to program success because they must support the sophisticated data entry systems necessary to fulfill reimbursement requirements for documentation, billing, and statistical record keeping. Management and supervisory staff also must be able to follow stringent federal and state regulatory requirements in addition to meeting the Joint Commission on Accreditation of Healthcare Organizations' rigorous standards.

Recruitment of appropriate and qualified clinical and operational staff for home care often is a barrier to providing services. The local supply of "home-grown" professionals committed to the hometown hospital is invariably insufficient to meet local or regional demand. Recent graduates and newcomers to the area usually are attracted to more traditional jobs in hospitals and clinics. Hospital and home care recruiters may find themselves competing for top candidates. Sparks can fly if the home care department is perceived to be luring away talent the hospital has worked long and hard to train and develop. Such conflicts may quickly spoil the environment for coordinated service delivery. Further, recruitment programs themselves may be imbedded in the inpatient culture, so newly hired staff frequently have no home health experience.

Geographical Barriers

A third barrier to rural case management is the large and often isolated service area most rural home health agencies must cover. Home care field staff must be prepared 24 hours a day, 7 days a week to travel many miles, often on isolated, unpaved roads and under hazardous weather conditions. A roadside search of the typical field staff car in the wintertime probably would turn up a large bag of salt, a shovel, blankets, a flashlight, candles, and granola bars.

Communication, without the benefit of phone equipment in many patient homes, presents a major difficulty for practitioners who need to notify their office or a physician's office regarding patient problems, emergencies, patients' conditions, or schedule changes. Car phones or portable cellular phones have remedied these situations for some providers. The field staff's travel expenses, disruptive calls, unscheduled stops, and the significant amount of unproductive travel time also are additional geographical barriers.

Ancillary and Support Service and Resource Barriers

Perhaps the most significant obstacle to providing effective home care services in rural areas is the dearth of supportive and ancillary services and important resources. Many rural home care agencies are unable to provide basic pediatric, psychiatric, or respiratory home care, for example. Due in part to the scarcity of qualified staff, inability to provide these vital services also may stem from lack of local physician expertise or interest, insufficient equipment and supplies, or inadequate education and training programs. Additionally, there may be a lack of hospital support for these services considering the small numbers of potential referrals.

Insufficient numbers of primary and subspecialty physicians in some areas may prompt patients and families to seek medical services in tertiary hospitals as far away as 200 miles. Spanning such great distances further complicates the inpatient discharge planning process for home care services. Discharge planning to home health care grows more inefficient with every mile, delaying physician review and approval of the treatment plan, physician-nurse consultations, and interagency communication. More important, the distance factor further interferes in the continuum of care for patients, families, and staff.

Another hindrance to discharge planning in rural areas is the unavailability of transportation to various social service agencies, support groups, and physicians' offices for follow-up medical care. In more remote areas, there are few if any resources for durable medical equipment, pharmaceuticals, and the newer technologies such as infusion therapy programs that are often required in a comprehensive home care treatment plan.

• Rural Home Health Case Management

Overcoming such imposing barriers will require aggressive action and sharp focus. As hospital-based home care continues to grow, hospitals must accept accountability for establishing programs that enhance access, promote high-quality patient care, and control costs. At Illinois Valley Community Hospital, formal programming efforts are led by a multidisciplinary team and daily operations are coordinated by an individual dedicated solely to that task.

The Case Management Coordinator Position

In the development of the case management coordinator position, it is crucial to involve hospital administration, discharge planners, home health management and staff, as well as the home health medical director. This collaborative approach will foster the participatory responsibility and accountability required for this unique position and will ensure the identification of a broad spectrum of issues that need to be addressed. A multidisciplinary team approach will facilitate a sense of project ownership, thus enhancing its success.

The written job description should specify performance standards and clinical and administrative qualifications for the position. A qualified case management coordinator would be a registered nurse, ideally holding a bachelor's degree, who has worked in both acute and home care settings. Determining candidates' knowledge of rural health systems and the barriers to home care service delivery in rural settings should be fundamental objectives of the recruitment and hiring process.

The Role of the Case Management Coordinator

The primary responsibility of the case management coordinator is to accept and initiate appropriate and timely patient referrals with a secondary obligation to negotiate care and reimbursement with third-party payers. A third level of accountability (although more subtle and having no less impact) is to become the home care liaison within the hospital and in the community. In this capacity, the case management coordinator assesses the barriers to providing home care and identifies and prioritizes efforts to overcome those barriers.

• Innovative Staffing Strategies

Staffing requires thoughtful planning from home care administration and commitment from hospital administration. Additionally, the case management coordinator must work with the hospital personnel and marketing and public relations departments along with the home health agency to devise tactics to recruit key home health personnel. Realistic and innovative programs such as weekend and supplemental staffing are paramount to program success. Through these programs, all interested hospital staff and others are given the opportunity to become involved in home care without leaving their current positions. This tactic also provides home care supervisors the opportunity to observe job performance before offering an individual a permanent position.

To facilitate future staff recruitment, the case management coordinator would do well to work closely with junior colleges and universities that feed health care professionals into the regional system. Home care agencies may offer mentorships and preceptorships at the baccalaureate and master levels, along with special programs for the associate degree students. Health care students and educators value the training and experience that home care offers. Of course, the case management coordinator also should work closely with various hospital departments to ensure ongoing communication, resource allocation, and inservicing in order to facilitate staff transfers to the home care department.

• Reduction of Philosophical and Operational Differences

The philosophical and operational differences between the hospital and its home care counterpart are conspicuous. The case management coordinator can assist hospital personnel to interpret home health policy and procedure, and vice versa. Case managers will be particularly effective in fulfilling this role if they participate on several hospital as well as home health committees.

Further, the case management coordinator is responsible for educating physicians concerning home health philosophies, capabilities, and referral processes. This includes discussing available home care services and interpreting home care policies and procedures and state and federal regulatory requirements for home care treatment plans and record maintenance. Fully informed physicians will embrace home care as a welcome complement to their practice. Once physicians and hospital administrative staff together understand the philosophy and operations of the home care department, their more cohesive thinking and synergistic planning efforts will benefit patients, providers, physicians, and payers alike.

• Deployment of the Troops

Illinois Valley Community Hospital's case management coordinator, working closely with the home health quality management coordinator and field staff supervisor, has divided the home care service area into four pie-shaped districts and assigned to each a home health team consisting of registered nurses, a licensed practical nurse, certified nurse assistants, and contractual physical, speech, and occupational therapists. The four teams share two social workers.

Team members are assigned to cases based on the level of their expertise and their proximity to the patients' homes. Basic agency policies and procedures guide the teams in standards of care, treatment plans, documentation, referral systems, and reimbursement requirements. The case management coordinator frequently interprets home care policies and procedures in light of the basic differences between inpatient and home care requirements.

• Ancillary and Support Services

Rural hospital-based home care agencies address the need for ancillary and support services in a variety of ways. The case management coordinator must develop close working relationships with both local and tertiary hospital discharge planners, physicians, and social service departments. This strategy allows hospital staff and home care case managers to identify patients' needs prior to discharge, confirm the best allocation of resources to meet those needs, and optimize the continuum of care for every patient. Further, it allows hospital and home care case managers to work closely with attending physicians in establishing appropriate and timely referral and discharge treatment plans.

The case management coordinator enhances the planning process and assists in reducing inpatient lengths of stay by bringing various disciplines together to address patients' posthospital needs and by facilitating earlier planning for home care.

• Resource Manuals

Practitioners in the field need a practical and quick reference to various social service agencies and local service providers. A resource manual can be assembled over time by the case management coordinator, based on their growing familiarity with other home health agencies, discharge planners from tertiary hospitals, local community agencies, and various other services and resources. Patients in remote rural areas often must seek access to medical care and services in urban areas. These referrals, too, can be simplified by an organized, exhaustive resource manual. Routinely refined and updated with appropriate information and phone numbers, the manual will soon prove invaluable to practitioners and case managers, allowing them to quickly and easily match patients' needs with the most appropriate services available in the service area.

• Measures of Success

The potential financial benefit of Illinois Valley Community Hospital's outpatient case management program is evident in its growing bottom-line contributions and visit volumes. During the first 18 months home care experienced a 35 percent increase in visits. Initially contributing only 1 to 3 percent of the hospital's bottom line, recent figures indicate that, with a continued growth in visit volume, home care may be expected to account for as much as 9 to 12 percent of the hospital's bottom line. The case management coordinator position plays a key role in this growth.

• Conclusion

Hospital-based home care departments already have been instrumental in enhancing the allocation of resources and delivery of care to the nation's rural population. As the health care system changes and rural health care becomes even more regionalized, the challenge will be to develop organized systems that can transcend the barriers to providing high-quality home care across great distances.

The future success of hospital-based home care departments will depend on the collaboration and cooperation of hospital administrators, home care administrations, and local community resources. Home care case managers and tertiary facility staff likewise must communicate and integrate their efforts to provide a continuum of care in the oftentimes difficult and always challenging rural environment.

Chapter 13

Case Management Model: Workers' Compensation

Patricia Alario

• Introduction

Employers today are taking a proactive role in curtailing the rising cost of workers' compensation benefits. In an economy where health care benefit costs represent nearly one-third of American companies' total profits, many employers are protecting their investment by utilizing case management to ensure high-quality health care while controlling costs.

Case management is a systematic approach to identifying high-cost patients, assessing the potential opportunities to coordinate their care, developing treatment plans that improve quality and control costs, and managing patients' total care to ensure optimum outcomes.[1] The historical roots of labor-based case management can be traced to the rehabilitation-based models that have been in use for workers' compensation cases since the 1940s.[2] More and more employers are turning to occupational health programs for effective workers' compensation case management. This chapter discusses how the occupational health nurse in the role of case manager works with the employer to provide an effective case management program.

• The Occupational Health Nurse as Case Manager

The occupational health case manager (almost always the occupational health nurse) must perform a number of primary functions. These include:[3]

- Assess the employee's and employer's needs
- Develop and implement a plan of care
- Make referrals to and collaborate with other health care providers
- Serve as liaison among employer, physician, employee, insurance company, and other allied health professionals
- Act as patient advocate

- Provide ongoing monitoring and coordination of treatment
- Plan and implement the return-to-work process
- Evaluate care outcomes

In essence, this case management model is merely an expansion of the traditional occupational health nursing process. With their background in acute care, their familiarity with standard courses of treatment, their knowledge of community resources, and their experience in coordinating workers' compensation cases, occupational health nurses are uniquely qualified to be case managers.

Despite all efforts toward prevention, work-related injuries and illnesses do occur. Early intervention and early return to work of the injured worker is one strategy to reduce lost work time, reduce disability, and lower medical costs. The case management of work-related injuries is a four-step process.

Step 1. The employer contacts the occupational health nurse as soon as he or she is aware that an injury has occurred. The case manager interviews the newly injured worker to ascertain a history of the injury and to gain an understanding of the job and the factors that may have contributed to the worker's injury. The case manager also notes any physical problems, emotional stressors, financial or family problems, and other barriers to improving the employee's health and ensuring his or her return to work. From the beginning, the case manager develops a therapeutic relationship with the injured employee and creates an expectation that the employee will return to work as soon as possible.

Step 2. The case manager develops and implements a plan of care in consultation with other members of the multidisciplinary health care team (physicians, physical therapists, occupational therapists, social workers, and counselors) and determines what services are necessary and the most cost-effective way to provide the needed care. The case manager does not usurp the role of the attending physician but, rather, reviews the patient's situation based on familiarity with standard courses of treatment and, if necessary, makes suggestions about treatment alternatives. Physician cooperation is an essential part of the case management process.

Step 3. The case manager acts as liaison among the employee, the insurance company, the employer, the physician, and the attorney (if one is involved). The case manager is responsible for timely and frequent communication among team members and keeps the company contact informed of the employee's progress. The case manager also takes an active role in making recommendations to management to eliminate factors that contributed to the injury.

Step 4. The case manager, again in collaboration with the multidisciplinary team, plans and implements the return-to-work process. One way for an employer to minimize workers' compensation costs is to develop a modified/alternate duty program. *Alternate duty* is a rehabilitation concept that mitigates the psychosocial aspects of disability by returning the disabled employee to a manageable level of productive work as early as possible. Alternate duty assignments disallow malingering and prevent total loss of productive hours for the employer. Even an employee with a back injury can work under controlled circumstances.

Employers frequently have contracts or agreements with local emergency departments (EDs) for managing the acute phase of injury—to provide diagnostic X rays, sutures, pain control, and so on. Emergency physicians and providers must understand the program goals for the injured worker, emphasizing the need for appropriate treatment and recommending alternate duty so that minimal time is lost in follow-up and rehabilitation care. Emergency physicians' awareness of the case management program's goals is elemental to cost containment efforts.

• The Return-to-Work Process

The return-to-work process involves a number of steps. These include having written policies in place, requirements for medical documentation, transitional return-to-work programs, and methods for managing the risks of prolonged disability.

Return-to-Work Policies

The company should have a written policy regarding the return-to-work process. Such a policy might wisely stipulate criteria such as the following:

- That the program will cover only employees with temporary work-related injuries and illnesses
- That alternate duty will be considered only when the employee can safely return to work without aggravating his or her injury
- That the employee and supervisor must adhere to the physician's medical restrictions to avoid aggravating the employee's condition
- That employees on alternate duty will be allowed to continue any necessary therapy and be paid their normal wage, which usually exceeds workers' compensation, to encourage a speedy return to work

In following the company's policy and coordinating the alternate duty program to return the injured employee to work, it is the case manager's responsibility to assure the employee and the physician that returning to work will not interfere with the employee's medical treatment.[4] The case manager communicates with the employee, the physician, and the company and obtains a written job description of the employee's usual activities. The case manager should then visit the work site to understand the employee's usual job and to identify specific alternate duties that the employee can safely perform with certain accommodations. Once the employee has returned to work on an alternate duty, the case manager maintains contact with the employee to resolve any problems that may arise.

Medical Documentation Requirements

The potential liability for returning an injured employee to work prematurely and possibly causing reinjury can be costly. Thus, great care must be taken to maintain detailed documentation of the return-to-work process and progression. The physician should document the specific restrictions (for example, no lifting over five pounds, no repetitive wrist motion, no bending or twisting at the waist) necessary for the employee to return to work on alternate duty and how long those restrictions will be in effect. This documentation enables the company to decide whether it can provide the necessary accommodations.

Transitional Return-to-Work Program

When an employee has been out of work for a long time, the case manager may recommend a transitional return-to-work program such as work hardening. *Work hardening,* traditionally performed by physical therapists, simulates a modified work program to improve the employee's functional capacity before returning to the workplace. Work hardening parallels work-related tasks but through graduated progression, education, and medical surveillance.[5]

Methods for Managing the Risks of Prolonged Disability

Comprehensive case management offers every opportunity to coordinate rehabilitation to effect an early return to work and avoid the substantial financial loss incurred as a result of prolonged disability. But statistics reveal that only 50 percent of workers return to their jobs after a work loss of six months or more; only 25 percent return to work after one year; and, after two years, the chance that a disabled employee will return to previous employment approaches zero.[6] When a disabled employee fails to return to work, medical problems often are compounded by psychosocial needs. In every case of prolonged disability, therefore, the case manager and other members of the health care team need to address the psychosocial aspects of disability.

A comprehensive psychosocial assessment begins with identification of certain factors related to disability; for example, depression, fear, lack of motivation, decreased self-esteem, substance abuse, poor coping mechanisms, pain management problems, and family stressors. The case manager should consider appropriate referrals for the evaluation and treatment of all employees unable to return to work for prolonged periods.[7]

Some employees may feel unable to return to work despite clearance from their physician. In such instances, the case manager should schedule an independent medical evaluation to clarify the employee's impairments or disabilities. This evaluation may result in a discontinuance of workers' compensation benefits.

• The Expanding Role of the Workers' Compensation Case Manager

Considering their central role in the delivery of health care for disabled workers, case managers are finding that their responsibilities are rapidly expanding to include quality assurance, health promotion, and prevention of illness/injury in the workplace. Evaluating the appropriateness of treatment, monitoring the patient's adherence to the treatment regimen, and ensuring that the employee's medical and psychosocial needs are met are increasingly vital functions of the workers' compensation case manager. These quality assurance measures provide essential feedback through which patient care can be monitored and improved.

Similar to other specialties in health care, occupational health has expanded its focus from simply treating injuries and illnesses to promoting health and the prevention of illness and injury in the workplace. In a holistic approach to workers' compensation and occupational health, the case manager assesses the condition of the workplace, identifies any health hazards, and works with the employer to eliminate or control those hazards. The workplace assessment also can assist employees in performing their tasks more ergonomically. Without such preventive measures, employees may be at continuous risk for work-related injury and illness, making even the most earnest efforts toward cost containment difficult to realize.

The case manager also may perform preplacement physical examinations to assist the employer in assessing new employees' ability to safely perform essential job functions. Without divulging specific diagnoses, the case manager notifies the employer of any limitations or reasonable accommodations that will be necessary in order for the employee to safely perform his or her job. This protects the employee from being placed in a position that could jeopardize his or her health and increase workers' compensation costs.

Both the company and its employees benefit when individuals adopt and maintain healthy life-styles. Employees' physical and mental health directly affects their productivity, and one way for employers to encourage healthier behavior is to provide screening and education programs, such as back injury prevention, in all areas of health and safety. For employers, health promotion yields many indirect benefits, such as decreased absenteeism, increased productivity, and lower turnover rates, and can have a direct impact on health care and workers' compensation costs.[8]

• Conclusion

With the occupational health nurse in the role of case manager, the workers' compensation case management model is built on the strongest of foundations. Occupational health nurses are uniquely qualified to work closely with other professional disciplines in coordinating the care of injured or disabled employees and arranging their timely return to the workplace. The case manager's understanding of the work environment fosters a holistic approach to case management that benefits both employee and employer. The further expansion of this case management model to include quality assurance and health promotion and wellness holds great promise for the future delivery of excellent health care in the nation's workplaces.

References

1. Conbere, P., McGovern, P., Kochevar, L., and Widtfeldt, A. Measuring satisfaction with medical case management. *AAOHN* 40(7):333–41, July 1992.

2. Henderson, M. G., and Collard A. Measuring quality in medical case management programs. *Quality Review Bulletin* 14(2):33–39, Feb. 1988.

3. National Association for Home Care. *Caring* 6(12):4–7, 34–44, Dec. 1987.

4. Dolney, W. Restricted work-activity programs minimize injury compensation costs. *Occupational Health & Safety* 61(6):75, 89, June 1992.

5. Bruyere, S., and Shrey, D. Disability management in industry: a joint labor–management process. *Rehabilitation Counseling Bulletin* 34(3):227–42, Mar. 1991.

6. Blum, A., and Mauch, R. RN case manager can help provide appropriate care, cost management. *Occupational Health & Safety* 59(4):68–69, Apr. 1990.

7. Greenwood, J., Wolf, H., Pearson, J., Woon, C., Posey, P., and Main, C. Early intervention in low back disability among coal miners in West Virginia: negative findings. *Journal of Occupational Medicine* 32(10):1047–52, Oct. 1990.

8. O'Brien, R. Managing health care quality can lower costs and generate access. *Benefits Quarterly* 7(4):17–22, Fourth Quarter 1991.

Bibliography

Blum, A., and Mauch, R. RN case manager can help provide appropriate care, cost management. *Occupational Health & Safety* 59(4):68–69, Apr. 1990.

Bruyere, S., and Shrey, D. Disability management in industry: a joint labor–management process. *Rehabilitation Counseling Bulletin* 34(3):227–42, Mar. 1991.

Conbere, P., McGovern, P., Kochevar, L., and Widtfeldt, A. Measuring satisfaction with medical case management. *AAOHN* 40(7):333–41, July 1992.

Cronin, C., and Maklebust, J. Case-managed care: capitalizing on the CNS. *Nursing Management* 20(3):38–47, Mar. 1989.

Dolney, W. Restricted work-activity programs minimize injury compensation costs. *Occupational Health & Safety* 61(6):75, 89, June 1992.

Eubanks, P. Case management and safety can cut workers' comp. *Hospitals* 64(6):80–81, Mar. 20, 1990.

Faherty, B. Case management the latest buzzword. *Caring* 9(7):20–22, July 1990.

Feeler, L. Task-specific rehab program reduces claims. *Occupational Health & Safety* 61(8):22–24, Aug. 1992.

Greenwood, J., Wolf, H., Pearson, J., Woon, C., Posey, P., and Main, C. Early intervention in low back disability among coal miners in West Virginia: negative findings. *Journal of Occupational Medicine* 32(10):1047–52, Oct. 1990.

Henderson, M., and Collard, A. Measuring quality in medical case management. *Quality Review Bulletin* 14(2):33–39, Feb. 1988.

Hereford, R. W. Private-pay case management. *Caring* 9(8):8–12, Aug. 1990.

Kantor, A. New role for nurses: tending to the bottom line. *Business and Health* 9(13):62–64, Dec. 1991.

Kemp, B. The case management model of human service delivery. *Annual Review of Rehabilitation* 2:212–38, 1981.

Levy, B., and Wegman, D. *Occupational Health Recognizing and Preventing Work-Related Disease.* Boston: Little, Brown and Co., 1988.

Mullahy, C. Cutting healthcare costs with case management. *Personnel* 66(9):50–51, Sept. 1989.

National Association for Home Care. *Caring* 6(12):4–7, 34–44, Dec. 1987.

Norris, M., and Hill, C. The clinical nurse specialist: developing the case manager role. *Dimensions of Critical Care Nursing* 10(6):346–53, Nov.–Dec. 1991.

O'Brien, R. Managing health care quality can lower costs and generate access. *Benefits Quarterly* 7(4):17–22, Fourth Quarter 1991.

Parry, A. E. How to tighten the reins on workers' compensation costs. *Healthcare Financial Management* 44(5):109–10, May 1990.

Pierog, L. Case management: a product line. *Nursing Administration Quarterly* 15(2):16–20, Winter 1991.

Schroer, K. Case management: clinical nurse specialist and nurse practitioner, converging roles. *Clinical Nurse Specialist* 5(4):189–94, 1991.

Schull, D., Tosch, P., and Wood, M. Clinical nurse specialists as collaborative care managers. *Nursing Management* 23(3):30–33, Mar. 1992.

Skagen, A. Managing healthcare costs, part 3: focus on case management. *Compensation and Benefits Review* 20(6):56–63, Nov.-Dec. 1988.

Smith, M. Individual case management: a win-win proposition. *Caring* 9(8):26–28, Aug. 1990.

Spann, K. Can workers' compensation be a cost savings? *Journal of Nursing Administration* 20(4):6, Apr. 1990.

Chapter 14

Case Management Model: Employee Assistance

Kathryn Cantey Church

• Introduction

Statistics show that employers bear the brunt of escalating health care costs in insurance premiums and workers' compensation fees. Over the past six years, U.S. corporations have spent as much on health care benefits as they have earned in after-tax profits. Left for the most part to their own resources, companies have been doing whatever they can to control costs and rein in spending.

Stress in the workplace can cause accidents and ailments such as ulcers, migraines, and heart disease, and employers spend billions of dollars every year to cover the resulting health care, absenteeism, and turnover costs. However, employers are beginning to learn that they can approach this problem by establishing employee assistance programs (EAPs).

The EAP case management model is a comprehensive health management strategy built on health promotion, prevention, and service coordination. Employee assistance professionals bring a comprehensive array of services directly to the work site. Designed to help identify and resolve health, work performance, and conduct problems and to address their underlying causes in employees' personal or family life, EAPs provide the direction and support that employees need to achieve a healthier life-style, modify harmful behaviors, improve productivity, and return to work earlier. This chapter describes how employee assistance programs can be successfully implemented to reduce disruption in the workplace caused by employee health or emotional disorders and to curb the employer's health care costs.

Ms. Church's views do not necessarily reflect those of the U.S. Office of Personnel Management.

• Health Management

Employee assistance programs were developed to identify and help employees resolve financial, relationship, drug or alcohol dependency, and other personal or family problems *before* they interfere with productivity, health, and job performance. Should the situation require a leave from work, the EAP monitors the employee's progress, ensures appropriate treatment, and manages his or her return to the workplace. Facilitating a smooth transition back to work may involve modifying the employee's work schedule and job responsibilities, in close coordination with his or her supervisors and coworkers. Some programs have even expanded to include employee problems for which there is little evidence of significant deterioration of work performance — for example, eldercare and child care responsibilities.[1]

Many EAPs also focus on wellness promotion as a means of prevention. Their efforts include offering seminars and individual programs on behavioral health care issues such as parenting, stress management, and dual-career management, as well as other health topics such as smoking cessation and nutrition maintenance.

• Program Background and Development

Employee assistance programs date back to the late 1800s, though the name was coined more recently and the current model has evolved over the past 20 to 25 years in both the private and public sectors. In 1985, Roman and Blum defined the *core technology* of EAPs that set the field apart from any other.[2] Of the six components that make up that core technology, two define an EAP's responsibilities in terms of case management. The first of these two definitions, "micro-linkages with counseling, treatment, and other community resources,"[3] refers to the responsibility of managing each individual case and includes the usage of external (to the organization) resources. The second definition, "the creation and maintenance of macro-linkages between the work organization and counseling, treatment, and other community resources,"[4] involves developing a better understanding between work organizations and community resources.

• The Role of Case Manager

To successfully implement the microlinkage component, employee assistance practitioners/case managers must fully understand both the internal and external resources that are available to them. Armed with current and relevant information about benefit plans and other employee programs available within the organization (for example, health promotion, wellness programs, retraining facilities, and career counseling/outplacement services), the EAP can put together the "best fit" for each individual employee. As with other case management efforts, resources and applications are individualized according to patient needs. External resources such as self-help programs, behavioral health programs, addiction treatment services, and legal options must be carefully managed to balance the needs of the employee, the employer, the payer, and the treatment program.

Microlinkages depend on the employee assistance case manager's ability to appropriately assess the employee's condition and needs and then to make an appropriate referral. The case manager must objectively administer each referral to the satisfaction of the referral source, the client, and the recipient of the referral, all within the payer's confines.

Macrolinkages require the case manager to track most clients throughout their course of treatment to gauge the effectiveness of the referral. Unfortunately, this essential outreach component of the case management process frequently is neglected because it is so labor-intensive.

The first step in developing macrolinkages is to develop a plan for evaluating all referral resources. Through their personal contacts employee assistance practitioners can assess the skills, philosophy, and atmosphere of referral sources and, conversely, can provide the referral source a better understanding of the employee's work organization. The case management process is enhanced with every successful referral that provides feedback and benefit to both employer and employee.

Follow-up after the referral is an important component of the EAP's responsibilities. Appropriate and well-established macrolinkages will ensure that a thorough follow-up is possible. Information obtained in the follow-up often is invaluable in assisting the employee to improve his or her work performance. Follow-up activities over the long term also provide valuable information about whether the system is really working, and that information may be instrumental in obtaining more appropriate benefits or in strengthening the case management process.

• Program Benefits

An effective employee assistance program yields several important benefits for providers, work organizations, and employees. The potential value of EAPs in terms of cost savings is inestimable. Direct revenue savings are realized in reduced health care costs, improved productivity, lower disability wages, and less absenteeism and turnover. The macrolinkage component of the model described above also creates an informal but effective network for employee assistance referrals and treatment linkages. Some EAPs now also provide a formal gatekeeping function or earmark a portion of the work organization's benefits dollars for employee behavioral health. More and more companies are coming to realize that EAPs are in the best position to evaluate their alternatives for cost-effective employee health care.

The case management components of EAPs have not yet been isolated to show their cost-effectiveness for work organizations, but EAPs clearly are working for both employees and organizations across the nation. Employees who are unable to rely on an EAP might instead approach their managers/supervisors for assistance with personal problems, taking those managers away from their own important duties and responsibilities. With a dedicated program available for both consultation and referral, managers can simply refer the employee to qualified professionals who are better able to help. Employees seem better able to concentrate on their jobs when they realize that professional assistance is available through their EAP.

Referral resources also benefit from the employee assistance program. The client referrals they receive from EAPs have already been evaluated by a qualified case manager who also provides (with the employee's signed release) valuable information regarding the employee's behavior or performance at work. (Note: Ethical guidelines prohibit employee assistance practitioners from referring clients to programs or practices they own and from receiving kickbacks for referrals.)

• Marketing and Education

Informing all employees that the EAP exists and explaining how it works are essential components of the program. Promotional materials (brochures, wallet cards, and so on), health promotion seminars, and supervisory training are a good start. The still unconvinced may demand more solid information. Analyses of program utilization and penetration and the performance of program alumni will demonstrate the EAP's effectiveness. The program also must continuously assess the treatment effectiveness and outcomes of its referral resources.

But perhaps the most effective marketing tool is the employee grapevine. After all is said and done, client satisfaction is the ultimate measure of a successful program.

• Conclusion

Employee assistance programs provide consultation, assessment, and referral services to treat a wide range of health and behavioral disorders that might otherwise severely disrupt the workplace. Besides coordinating traditional services, EAP case managers may develop and implement comprehensive educational programs, including seminars, large group lectures, publications, and management training.

Employers have been swift to embrace the EAP concept in their ongoing efforts to curb rising health care costs. Nipping potentially disastrous personal and organizational situations in the bud and offering just the right resources directly to the people who need them, EAPs have turned out to be a wise investment of scarce health care dollars.

References

1. Erfurt, J. C., Foote, A., and Heirich, M. A. Integrating employee assistance and wellness: current and future core technologies of a megabrush program. *Journal of Employee Assistance Research* 1(1):1–31, Summer 1992.

2. Roman, P. M., and Blum, T. C. The core technology of employee assistance programs. *The ALMACAN* 15(3):8–19, Mar. 1985.

3. Roman and Blum.

4. Roman and Blum.

Bibliography

Blum, T. C., Martin, J. K., and Roman, P. M. A research note on EAP prevalence, components and utilization. *Journal of Employee Assistance Research* 1(1):209–29, Summer 1992.

Dickman, F., Challenger, B. R., Emener, W. G., and Hutchison, W. S., Jr. *Employee Assistance Programs*. Springfield, IL: Charles C. Thomas, 1988.

Erfurt, J. C., Foote, A., and Heirich, M. A. Integrating employee assistance and wellness: current and future core technologies of a megabrush program. *Journal of Employee Assistance Research* 1(1):1–31, Summer 1992.

Johnson, R. B., and Malone, E. Building an integrated EAP–MBHC program: the preferred provider network. *EAPA Exchange* 22(11):41–43, Nov.–Dec. 1992.

Lewis, J. A., and Lewis, M. D. *Counseling Programs for Employees in the Workplace*. Monterey, CA: Brooks/Cole Publishing Co., 1986.

Roman, P. M., and Blum, T. C. The core technology of employee assistance programs. *The ALMACAN* 15(3):8–19, Mar. 1985.

Wenzel, L. Effective case systems integrate costs and service needs. *Occupational Health & Safety* 4(3):37–41, 72, Apr. 1988.

Chapter 15

Case Management Model: Perinatal and Neonatal Services

Patricia DeHof

• Introduction

Perinatal and neonatal home care services are particularly well suited to the outpatient case management concept. *Perinatal home care*—provided to mothers before and shortly after childbirth—offers optimum health care for the high-risk mother and significant cost savings for the payer by reducing the incidence of premature birth, eliminating its attendant clinical problems and costs. *Neonatal home care*—provided to newborns—allows both mothers and babies to be discharged from acute care facilities much earlier, significantly reducing costly lengths of stay.

Because the expense of providing these preventive outpatient alternatives is so easily offset by real cost savings and excellent clinical outcomes, organized case management for perinatal and neonatal outpatient services is gaining wide acceptance. Both hospitals and special home health programs are responding to marketplace dynamics with new programs to meet consumer and payer needs. Caremark Women's Health, a specialized home health agency in Columbia, Maryland, employs a case management model that meets the growing demand for home perinatal and neonatal services in its market, while keeping a sharp eye on cost and quality. The Caremark model places its case managers—the agency's professional home care nurses—directly at the care site. Led in their care planning and actions by the referring physician, these home care nurses are supremely qualified to provide sound case management.

This chapter describes the advantage of the perinatal and neonatal case management model as experienced by providers, payers, and patients. Additionally, it uses the program at Caremark Women's Health to illustrate how these case management services might be developed and marketed to physicians, nurses, and payers.

• The Shift to Home Care

In the recent past, perinatal services were delivered primarily in hospitals to patients confined to a high-risk antenatal, labor and delivery, or post-partum unit. Today, thanks to advances in technology and therapeutics, perinatal services can be safely delivered in the patient's home environment by highly skilled registered nurses (RNs). Monitoring systems that warn of preterm labor conditions and home infusion for tocolytic therapy are the two most frequently utilized perinatal outpatient procedures. Advances in telecommunications allow the immediate transport of patient monitoring data to remote locations, revolutionizing monitoring techniques in the out-patient environment.

Although all women experiencing a high-risk pregnancy may benefit from perinatal case management services, the majority of referrals are initiated by private physicians or insurance companies. The most common reasons for high-risk mothers to utilize monitored services are existing pre-term labor, a history of prior preterm labor and/or delivery of a preterm infant, and multiple gestation. Additional diagnoses that may require case management or home care include, but are not limited to, hyperemesis, gesta-tional diabetes, history of deep-vein thrombosis requiring heparin therapy, pregnancy-induced hypertension, and postpartum maternal child care.

Neonatal and postpartum home care programs also have emerged recently as a powerfully cost-effective means of reducing the length of new mothers' and newborns' hospital stays. It is not uncommon today for a mother to be encouraged to leave the hospital with her newborn within 6 to 24 hours after delivery. Should mother or infant require routine or spe-cial services, in-home assessment, health care education, and homemaker support are provided by an RN. Some hospital-based programs routinely provide a minimum of two postpartum visits for all first-time mothers and those participating in breast feeding.

Although employers and payers have been the driving force behind many such initiatives, home perinatal, neonatal, and postpartum care have become popular options among patients, who consider these services a valuable benefit that limits the disruption of the family unit and yields savings for both patient and payer.

• The Development and Marketing of Case Management Services

To become a successful provider of home perinatal and neonatal case management services, several elements are essential. From the beginning, a team representing various disciplines and with a background in high-risk pregnancy and neonatal care must be involved in the actual development of the program. Teamwork among the medical equipment and product line sales force and the clinicians is essential in the inception of this program. Sales and nursing personnel bring varied backgrounds to the table and, therefore, enrich each other's understanding of the start-up process.

To stack up against the intense competition in home perinatal/neonatal health care, the sales and nursing staffs at Caremark Women's Health have worked together as a team to develop the program and market its services to physicians, nurses, and payers. Prospective referral sources and clients even ask for a direct comparison with a competing program, so the team is always prepared for both clinical and financial questions. Caremark has found that physicians, nurses, and payers react more favorably toward the marketing team when both the sales and nursing staffs are in attendance during a presentation. Sales division representatives are best able to answer inquiries about cost and contracts with payers, and nurses can demonstrate a typical patient teaching session or answer questions regarding the actual care a patient may receive.

The marketing team still faces opposition to home care for the high-risk antepartum patient, which remains controversial in some circles. Conflicts among physicians, payers, and the home care provider will and do occur and must therefore be considered in the overall model for case management. One proven practice to reduce conflicts among these disciplines is direct and frequent communication. When a referral is phoned into the home care organization, it is essential that the health professional receiving the information understand the care plan and assure the referring physician that the program will provide the patient with the optimal care necessary to promote a good outcome. Taking time at the beginning of the referral process to outline a plan of care suitable to both the referring physician and the home care provider will decrease conflict during the treatment period. Depending on the therapy ordered, the physician may be contacted by the home care staff, the pharmacist, or the clinical nutritionist with updates regarding the patient's status and suggestions for continued home management.

This multidisciplinary team approach is essential for a satisfactory outcome for the home-based perinatal, postpartum, and neonatal client. Physicians generally welcome this approach to health care. During the sales presentation, the marketing team should stress that the home care organization must function as an extension of the physician's practice and not cause the "loss of control" that so many physicians find objectionable.

Quality control is an essential part of any health care organization. Periodic review of standard operating procedures as well as continuing education programs for staff members contribute to the overall quality of the home care provider and its personnel. Outcome criteria must be measurable and selected as a measure of excellence in order for a home-based health care organization to establish its niche in this marketplace. The endorsement and support of a large, nationally recognized corporation may be necessary in the early months for a novice in the women's health care arena, but as the agency's reputation as a leader in the perinatal home management field grows, it may rely on its own record as a provider of high-quality care.

• The Financial Incentives for Outpatient Case Management

Financial incentives for the home care perinatal client and payer are many and varied. The most apparent cost savings is simply the difference between costs incurred during an average hospital stay and the daily rate charged by an insurance company for home care of the same client. According to the National Association of Children's Hospitals and Related Institutions, the typical hospital cost for a premature infant weighing less than 5 pounds 8 ounces at birth was $67,533 in 1990. With an estimated 30,000 to 48,000 premature births during that year, total hospital costs multiplied to between $2 and $3.3 billion.[1] In sharp contrast, the entire cost of managing perinatal cases in the home is less than $250 per day over an average length of service of six weeks, generating a total cost of only $10,500 per case.

Home postpartum nursing has become more popular with the advent of short-stay maternity programs. Patients cared for in their own homes save obvious hospital costs; they also save in the cost of transportation to the hospital or outpatient facility, in lower child care costs, and in insurance copayments for those whose carriers require a copayment for every physician or health care facility visit. Other indirect cost savings arise from the elimination of hospital-based phone and television charges, on-road meals, and parking fees.

Payers also enjoy revenue savings by avoiding costly inpatient hospital stays, allowing them to maintain rather than increase their rates to the employers. Ultimately, the payer's savings are passed along to the consumer. As an incentive for physicians and patients to choose home care services, some insurance companies have included home care as a full benefit paying 100 percent of costs incurred, as compared to the 80/20 split they commonly pay for physician and hospital fees.

• Conclusion

Alternative sites (such as birthing centers) and shorter maternity stays are already revolutionizing the entire birthing process. Agency or hospital-based case management initiatives will continue to grow and evolve as the most economical alternative to acute care delivery. As more research and outcomes studies provide additional proof of the cost savings and quality benefits of in-home care for the mother, the unborn, and the neonate, services formerly reserved for the acute care setting will shift to the outpatient sector. New markets for technology and case management services will spring up as managed care contractors and others in the know attest to their safety and efficacy, and admissions criteria for in-home care management will soon relax as data confirm the safety of outpatient monitoring and innovative care delivery mechanisms. The many women and children who stand to benefit from this health care revolution will benefit all the more in perinatal and neonatal home care programs that employ sound case management strategies.

Reference

1. Brown, D. The siren song of a diagnostic test. *The Washington Post Health,* May 25, 1993, p. 11.

Chapter 16

Case Management Model: HIV/AIDS

Susan C. Rucker, Joel E. Abrams, and Margaret E. Piazza

• Introduction

Human immunodeficiency virus (HIV) infection today is increasingly viewed as a chronic, manageable illness. Over the past several years, as knowledge about and treatment of HIV/AIDS (acquired immune deficiency syndrome) have advanced, so has the medical management of HIV/AIDS clients in the outpatient setting. However, in the battle against this often debilitating illness and its psychosocial impact, the HIV/AIDS population is placing complex demands on medical, financial, and community resources.

The AIDS care program at Johns Hopkins Hospital provides education and offers recourse for families and individuals as they experience various stages of the disease process. The case management component creates a structured process that spans many disciplines, always focusing on the intricate health and social needs of patients. This focused approach makes available the most appropriate choice of therapies and care delivery sites, and coordinates the many supportive resources required to meet myriad medical, psychological, and social needs. This chapter describes the HIV/AIDS case management model at Johns Hopkins Hospital and discusses the benefits of such a program and the barriers to its implementation.

• Program Background

The Johns Hopkins University School of Medicine's AIDS Service, under a grant from the Maryland State AIDS Administration, piloted a model of coordinated assessment and case management for people infected with HIV, the virus most directly associated with AIDS. Named the Diagnostic Evaluation Unit (DEU), this model was intended to create a statewide system of community-based medical and case management services for people with HIV infection. Its primary objectives were the following:

- To guarantee every HIV-infected patient access to comprehensive, multi-disciplinary assessment and care planning
- To establish a linkage with ongoing medical and case management services
- To ensure compliance with various medical and treatment regimens to avoid the onset of opportunistic infection, reduce the potential for acute illness, and avoid costly hospital admission

Education also plays a major role in HIV/AIDS case management, considering that patient behavior modification may benefit the entire community by reducing the risk of HIV transmission.

One of the fundamental strategies in the pilot process was to identify various community resources willing and able to provide the services required. In addition, the pilot was intended to identify any significant service gaps that might create barriers to implementation and resource coordination. At present, the pilot phase of the DEU has ended and the AIDS Administration continues to move toward a fully integrated system of diagnostic assessment centers, medical care providers, and case management providers (such as county health departments, community service agencies, and drug treatment centers) throughout the state. The current goal of the DEU system is to provide continuity of care to all Maryland residents with HIV infection throughout the course of illness — from asymptomatic infection to full-blown AIDS. The program's primary objectives remain unchanged.

Although the Johns Hopkins DEU remains the single largest provider of HIV/AIDS assessment and medical services in Maryland, case management services in the community have expanded to meet the statewide demand created by the DEU system. This expansion of service is attributable to three factors:

1. The prior existence of private, not-for-profit, community-based HIV social service agencies in Baltimore (the most concentrated service population center)
2. The combined influence of the original pilot partners in establishing designated case managers within each county's local health department
3. The entry of an additional funding source through the Medical Assistance Targeted Case Management program, which provides monthly remuneration to participating programs for each individual Medical Assistance client served

Community medical services are further expanding as funds from various sources, such as Medical Assistance and Ryan White grants, become more widely dispersed.

• How the Model Works

In practical application, the model works as follows: A patient with an appointment for medical assessment in the Johns Hopkins HIV outpatient clinic (or the analogous clinics at other DEU sites) is asked to participate in a psychosocial assessment by a DEU social worker. Both the medical and psychosocial assessments have been standardized by the DEU. Patients who complete the assessment process then receive an individualized care plan formulated by a multidisciplinary team of designated DEU caregivers and social workers. On follow-up, the patient reviews the care plan with the DEU social worker and is given the option of being assigned a case manager based at a community agency or at the site of ongoing medical care.

Should the patient select case management, she or he is referred to the provider of choice, where case manager and patient together complete the care plan by identifying specific objectives to resolve the problems and goals identified by the assessment team. As mentioned earlier, if the patient is a Medical Assistance client, both the DEU and the case management agency may be eligible for individual reimbursement based on their agencies' participation in the program. Once a patient selects a case manager, that case manager is responsible for maintaining minimum monthly contact with the patient as well as for implementing the specific objectives of the care plan.

• Benefits of HIV/AIDS Case Management

For HIV/AIDS patients, the primary advantage of case management is the case manager's ability to act as a single point of contact to resolve myriad clinical and psychosocial issues. People with HIV place demands on virtually every form of social service, entitlement service, and community health service available. Indeed, the needs of people with HIV often outweigh the available resources. Case managers are able to guide patients to the proper resources, help them through the application processes required, and serve as advocates when a service delivery system is inadequate to meet patient needs.

Case managers assist community agencies to achieve efficient and fiscally responsible performance by monitoring patient eligibility for programs and assisting patients in correct program application, thus reducing the number of ineligible applicants requiring processing and avoiding costly duplication of services.

Additionally, case managers help patients maintain compliance with medical care and treatment regimens. Compliance with antiretroviral and prophylactic treatments among patients with HIV infection is proven to prevent or delay the onset of opportunistic infections and the resulting hospitalizations. Compliance also may reduce the severity of acute illness, thereby shortening the length of stay when hospitalization is unavoidable.

Finally, case managers provide ongoing education and instruction on transmission reduction behaviors and assist patients in maintaining compliance with new behaviors. As mentioned earlier, these preventive components can benefit the entire community by reducing the risk of further HIV transmission.

• Barriers to Program Implementation

A successful DEU system begins with an adequate number of participating community medical and case management providers who can allocate the proper human resources to staff the DEU assessment teams and create individualized care plans. A primary barrier in the Maryland DEU system has been a *lack of assessment teams capable of serving the volume of patients eligible for service.* The Johns Hopkins DEU, the only source of DEU services in the pilot phase and the largest ongoing DEU provider, operates in an outpatient clinic with a four- to six-month waiting period for new patient appointments. Because community clinics and providers capable of providing the necessary medical evaluation did not originally have the ability to perform psychosocial evaluations or convene multidisciplinary teams to write individual care plans, assessment soon became a bottleneck in the DEU process, delaying patient access to case management by months. Subsequent expansion of DEU assessment teams into other sites of primary and secondary HIV medical care has helped to open this bottleneck but has not eliminated it entirely.

Operational barriers for the system include *competition among case management organizations and the still-limited availability of HIV/AIDS-related services and resources.* Also, under current program regulations, the system becomes confusing when the primary case management agency—as specified in the individualized care plan—refers or discharges a patient to another community agency. For example, a patient case-managed through a drug treatment center may require the pro bono legal services of another agency in the DEU system. But under the DEU contract only the primary case management agency, the drug treatment center, is eligible for financial reimbursement for providing case management services; the referral agency is not reimbursed for any services it provides. Conversely, a discharge from the primary case management agency's direct service is considered a discharge from its case management services as well. Thus, a patient whose legal problems result in a discharge from the drug treatment center would lose her or his eligibility for case management by the drug treatment program. To transfer the case management to a new agency, the assessment team must reconvene and write a new care plan for the patient.

Inadequate social service resources pose the most serious operational barrier to case management. Inadequate transportation, child care, housing, finance, insurance, drug treatment, and legal services are all barriers for case managers trying to implement the care plan objectives. Fortunately, the collaborative nature of the DEU system creates avenues for creative interventions and an organized source of advocacy that sometimes fills these service gaps.

The DEU system involves a diverse range of professionals practicing within a variety of agencies. This need for collaboration highlights the importance of clearly defined roles, practice guidelines, and quality assurance measures. Successful program implementation requires the cooperation and willingness of the component agencies to change their usual patterns of sharing client information. The DEU experience illustrates the value of a comprehensive network that is accessible to all agencies and that identifies the client's activities within the participating community. However, it is not yet clear which agency can or should assume responsibility for establishing practice criteria, engaging community cooperation, or enforcing compliance.

The Diagnostic Evaluation Unit model of assessment and case management is one method of linking a wide variety of state, public, and private community health and social service providers in a structured, yet informal network capable of providing coordinated and continuous care to HIV-infected patients, while maintaining individual program autonomy. Although many barriers remain, the DEU has been a vital force in expanding service availability to a greater number of Maryland's HIV/AIDS population.

• A Case Study

The scenario in this section provides a personalized example of how the case management of an individual HIV-infected patient is assessed and implemented. The first part of the process is to obtain a patient profile.

The Client Profile

Sel is a 27-year-old African-American woman who presented to the outpatient HIV clinic on May 10, 1993. She was casually dressed and cooperative, with periods of tearfulness during the assessment interview. Accompanied by her 9 month old in a stroller and stating that her other child, an 8 year old, was in school, Sel was attentive to her baby and apparently comfortable talking with the social worker. Her medical history was unremarkable except for having had her tubes tied following an abortion 4 months ago. She stated that she did not want another "AIDS baby." Sel's younger child is followed in the Children's HIV Clinic, and Sel stated that she prays every day that he will not turn out to be HIV-positive.

Sel admits to a history of 10 years of injection use of heroin and cocaine and uses both intermittently now, between one and four times every couple of weeks. She claims that she wants to take good care of her baby and is trying "really hard" to curtail her drug use. She has had several detox experiences in the past. She does not use alcohol.

Medical evaluation reveals that Sel has thrush and is complaining of fatigue, some weight loss, and multiple recurrent bouts of vaginitis. Her T-cell count is 46.

Sel has an eleventh-grade education, and her longest period of employment was 5 months working in housekeeping in a large commercial office building. She lives with her children in a one-bedroom apartment and supports the family on income from Aid to Families with Dependent Children (AFDC); she receives $420 from AFDC and $90 in food stamps. In addition, she receives federal medical assistance for each member of the family.

The children's father is intermittently available for financial and parenting support. Sel has not told him about her or their child's HIV status, although he has been asking questions about the child's frequent hospital visits. Sel does not know if her partner has ever been tested for HIV. She states that her request that he use condoms during sex resulted in a blowup followed by several days of suspicious and accusatory remarks by him.

Sel's social support system is limited. Her family of origin includes her mother, who has chronic cardiac problems, and an older brother, who is incarcerated and also HIV-positive. Her father is deceased and her only other sibling, a younger sister, died from a drug overdose.

She has not disclosed her HIV status to any of her friends and has no connection with a church. Sel reports that she knows of no one in the family who has been treated for psychiatric illness, although her mother experiences periods of tearfulness and self-neglect. She reports that she herself has difficulty staying asleep, has decreased libido, poor appetite, and finds it "hard to get going in the morning." She reports previous periods in her life that were characterized by vegetative symptoms suggestive of major depression, but she admits she was actively using drugs during that time. During the interview she stated she was not experiencing homicidal or suicidal ideation.

Sel's Case Management

Sel identifies several problems with which she wants help. She wants to be admitted to a drug treatment program; she wants a larger apartment for her family; and she needs transportation to the clinic. The social worker identifies several other concerns regarding Sel's limited support and isolated life: the younger child's health status and the future for both children; Sel's frequent unavailability for parenting due to drug use; her possible continued exposure from/to her partner; her partner's possible reaction to disclosure; and her acceptance and understanding of the need to begin antiretroviral therapy, PCP prophylaxis, and psychiatric assessment.

Any meaningful discussion of Sel's case must begin with the overall goal of HIV case management. Harder + Kibbe point out a lack of clarity in the literature on this subject—some authors highlighting the administrative nature of case management and others espousing a supportive style. The primary goal of case management may be cost control, it may be client-centered with a quality of life focus, or its primary aim might be service coordination. Harder + Kibbe's review of the literature indicates that, no matter what their primary goal, most HIV case management programs emphasize one or more of the following:[1]

- Increasing quality of care and quality of life for persons with HIV and AIDS
- Improving service coordination, access, and delivery
- Reducing costs of care through coordinated services to keep persons with HIV and AIDS out of the hospital
- Providing client advocacy and crisis intervention services

The common components of HIV/AIDS case management include some form of assessment process with resource identification, development of a plan of action, linkage and coordination between and among involved parties, monitoring of future needs, and disengagement at some defined endpoint.[2-8] Throughout these activities, a range of interventions may occur with the patient alone or with the patient and some other component of the environment, for example, the spouse, a housing agency, and/or children.

In Sel's case, assessment has identified problems for initial action: drug use, thrush, vaginitis, and psychiatric assessment. Further assessment is indicated in several areas: clarifying the health status of the baby and Sel's relationship with the hospital on that issue, and exploration of the partner's blowup and the patient's risk for domestic violence. Assessing the adequacy of the physical environment and Sel's parenting needs may require a home visit.

The plan for Sel's care will have certain short-term goals (for example, to obtain needed medicines) and long-term goals (for example, to plan for the children's future) requiring ongoing assessment and a variety of program linkages. Referrals to psychiatric assessment and care, drug treatment, and rental subsidy programs should be made. The hospital staff in the pediatric AIDS program should be involved in order to better understand the child's situation and Sel's relationship with those professionals. It may be that hospital visits can be coordinated to eliminate multiple trips, if that is an appropriate goal, or to provide more visits if Sel finds frequent contact a support. Through this team approach, redundancies in service provision can be reduced and the case manager can better serve Sel's family's needs.

Sel's advocacy needs are not yet clarified. Certainly it may be necessary to advocate for a patient in certain arenas, such as with housing programs. The issue of safer sexual practices for Sel must be addressed at some point. That her partner does not know she has HIV is troubling, because he is at risk of infection from her. However, it must be remembered that Sel is the client and her interests are paramount. She has not informed her partner presumably for good reasons. The dynamic of their relationship needs to be understood before she is encouraged to disclose her HIV status to him. Her silence on this issue may well be protecting her, if not her children, from more immediate harm.

Monitoring this patient and her family needs is critical. It can be safely predicted that Sel will have new needs in the future. She may need a home aide to assist with household chores so that she can remain a vital part of her children's lives. Home care for the baby and for Sel may become realities that need to be coordinated. Engaging other family members who have been distant is certainly a priority in terms of providing social support, repairing relationships, and providing for the future needs of the unaffected child. Good case management can ensure accurate assessment and timely intervention as the patient's needs change.

• Conclusion

HIV/AIDS patients currently represent one of the fastest-growing markets in the entire outpatient sector, a resource-consumptive market that is experiencing mounting expenditures for cost of care, medications, housing, and other required support systems. The diverse and complex nature of this disease process, combined with its disregard for age, gender, and race, offers challenge heretofore unfamiliar to many health care organizations and their respective communities. The need for distinctive practice modalities and case management initiatives for this patient population is paramount to establishing community health and eventual cost containment initiatives.

References

1. Harder + Kibbe Research. Challenges for the future: coordinating HIV/AIDS care and services in the next decade. Report of the National Symposium on Case Management and HIV/AIDS submitted to Sierra Health Foundation, May 1992.

2. American Hospital Association. *Case Management: An Aid to Quality and Continuity of Care.* Chicago: AHA, 1987.

3. Bachrach, L. Case management: toward a shared definition. *Hospital and Community Psychiatry* 40(9):883–84, 1989.

4. Fariello, D., and Scheidt, S. Clinical case management of the dually diagnosed patient. *Hospital and Community Psychiatry* 40(10):1065–67, 1989.

5. Kanter, J. Clinical case management: definition, principles, components. *Hospital and Community Psychiatry* 40(4):361–68, 1989.

6. Mor, V., Piett, J., and Fleishman, J. Community-based case management for persons with AIDS. *Health Affairs,* Winter 1988, pp. 139–53.

7. Ryndes, T. The coalition model of case management for care of HIV-infected persons. *Quality Review Bulletin,* Jan. 1989, pp. 4–8.

8. Sonsel, G. Case management in a community based AIDS agency. *Quality Review Bulletin,* Jan. 1989, pp. 31–36.

Chapter 17

Case Management Model: Behavioral Health Services

Roger B. Upson, PhD

• Introduction

Behavioral health services, including mental health and chemical dependency, are an important and often difficult to manage part of many employers' benefits package. This chapter describes and evaluates the case management structure started by Health One Corporation, a multihospital organization in Minneapolis and St. Paul, and continued by its successor organization, HealthSpan Corporation. Health One established a preferred provider arrangement for behavioral health services for its employees and their dependents, and later extended it to other employee groups and payers. The arrangement includes inpatient, outpatient, and partial-day services in the organization's hospitals and directs ambulatory services through a network of psychiatrists, psychologists, and other behavioral health service professionals.

The whole preferred provider arrangement now involves four hospitals, about 60 psychiatrists, and approximately 160 other professional providers, and it operates on a managed fee-for-service basis. Hospital services are provided at a discount; other providers pay a percentage of their reimbursement to help cover the administrative costs of the arrangements, and employers are charged a per-employee fee.

Although the arrangement manages care across the continuum of service possibilities, more than 90 percent of the patients are treated as outpatients. Consequently, outpatient case management is a principal activity. This chapter describes the components and benefits of the behavioral health service case management model.

• Model Components

The behavioral health case management model has four functional components. These are:

1. A triage system
2. A physician advisory council
3. A medical director
4. A manager

The Triage System

At the heart of the model is a telephone triage system comprising several behavioral health professionals, mainly nurses, who provide 24-hour-a-day, 365-day-a-year case management service to subscribers. The triage system serves several important functions. First, it enables callers to get immediate professional service and referral into the most appropriate, least restrictive level of service and gives them a clear understanding of the applicable benefits available in their medical insurance plan. Second, triage provides a basis for case management, because providers are required to file a treatment plan. The triage staff review treatment plans, follow up on the care provided, and identify more complex cases, such as multiple members of a family receiving care or sequential series of treatments. Third, the triage process provides confidentiality for those who may wish to remain anonymous or be treated at a location neutral to where they live or work. Fourth, triage helps both the employer and the employee/dependent minimize their total costs by guiding the client in the right direction through a network of preferred providers. Directed care also generates the volume of business that employers and providers need to justify a network pricing approach.

Staffing for the triage system has evolved to include both full-time and part-time professionals. The infrastructure for the network includes both phone and computer support. The phone system involves a complex arrangement of fixed-site phones, mobile phones, and beepers to ensure that there are multiple levels of backup behind the first response triage person. This complexity is needed to meet the standards set by the physician advisory council—standards that reflect customer needs for a prompt response to every call. The computer system supports the tracking of cases, the scheduling of appointments, and the preprocessing of bills from providers.

The Physician Advisory Council

The physician advisory council, chaired by the medical director, includes psychiatrists representing areas such as mental health, substance abuse, and adolescent and adult services and a licensed consulting psychologist. The manager and selected other staff also attend council meetings.

The council's role is to provide clinical advice and leadership. Over the years, it has developed and/or approved treatment guidelines, case management protocols, and a system for ensuring that all nonpsychiatric providers have a collaborative supervisory agreement with one of the network psychiatrists, in order to provide continuous quality assessment and improvement across the network. From time to time, the medical members themselves review particularly complex cases. The council interviewed the initial triage staff and sets the standards for the triage service in terms such as speed of service and protocols to be followed. The council secured its own legal opinion on the arrangement's provider contracts so that it could recommend them to other providers. In addition, the council handles various other medical/administrative issues, such as writing the position description for the medical director; appointing subcommittees for credentialing, for example; and drafting rules related to undocumented days or failure to file timely treatment plans.

The Medical Director

The medical director is a part-time position, with responsibility for medical oversight of clinical services, utilization review, and case management. This includes facilitating peer reviews and case management reviews of both inpatient and outpatient cases.

The Manager

The manager of this preferred provider arrangement has both operating and marketing responsibilities. Operating responsibilities include product design and network access, pricing and utilization reporting, and quality assurance and utilization review. Product design and network access involves coordinating the network resources to provide the complete continuum of services in accessible locations. Pricing and utilization data are the basis for utilization reports to the physician advisory council and for pricing and aggregate utilization reporting to employers. Quality assurance and utilization review include implementation of the physician advisory council's guidelines and are a key part of managing the triage system.

• Program Benefits

From a patient perspective, the case management services provided by the triage staff facilitate the entire process of assessment, referral, and treatment. Because the staff work closely with the employee assistance program, employees find their care well coordinated, with less duplication of activity.

From a provider perspective, the arrangement has directed business to the network providers and has improved coordination of services. Arising from their cooperation in this arrangement, the physicians and hospital administrators have jointly developed a product line management approach for behavioral health services for the whole multihospital organization.

From a payer perspective, the arrangement has provided cost control and, based on the reduced frequency of complaints about how behavioral health services are provided, has improved employee satisfaction. The arrangement has brought some control to an area that was previously unmanaged and where subscribers received no help in seeking care. It has enabled employers to provide guidance to employees, to obtain case management services that direct most cases to outpatient settings, and to avoid paying for expensive and nonregulated services.

• Conclusion

Built on a network of preferred providers, a leadership team of knowledgeable clinicians, and a responsive triage system staffed by trained professionals, this outpatient case management model for behavioral health services has yielded significant benefits for patients, providers, and payers alike. Case management has proven to be a highly effective way of coordinating these otherwise difficult-to-manage but vital outpatient services.

Chapter 18

Case Management Model: Chemical Dependency and Substance Abuse Treatment

Arthur M. Melvin

• Introduction

In recent years, sweeping clinical and economic changes have rocked the foundation of traditional substance abuse and chemical dependency treatment. The skyrocketing cost of treating substance abusers and chemical dependents has fueled higher insurance fees, patient copayments and deductibles, and has therefore reduced access to inpatient programs and limited coverage for outpatient care. Further, a lack of scientific outcome studies on treatment effectiveness has started turf struggles and ideological disagreements among competing disciplines, providers, and payers.

New concepts in outpatient case management have emerged to address the clinical and economic challenges of serving this special patient population. The goals of chemical dependency and substance abuse treatment are:

- To break the dependency syndrome
- To improve overall physical health and psychological functioning
- To restore employment and productivity
- To renew family life
- To develop educational/vocational skills
- To assist clients to assess their personal values

The case management model developed at Seton House, in Washington, DC, is designed to meet these goals and to help persons with multiple medical and social problems make the transition from institutionalized care to independent living. This chapter defines the role of the case manager in the chemical dependency and substance abuse treatment model, and describes the outpatient case management concept employed at Seton House.

• Model Components

At Seton House, the term *case management* refers to the coordination of individualized patient services and the utilization management component of optimal, cost-effective care. These case management responsibilities — care and cost — are divided between two groups: the program treatment staff who coordinate the entire clinical course of treatment, and the utilization review case managers who are responsible for cost containment. Authorized admission to an inpatient treatment center for chemical dependency requires certification by a health plan or entitlement program with inpatient care benefits. With these model components, Seton House can offer the service features so essential to program success: close supervision, supportive mechanisms, and compliance monitors integrated throughout a continuum of care.

• The Evolving Role of the Case Manager

Case management in addictions treatment traditionally referred only to the coordination of patient treatment planning. The general course of treatment for a privately insured patient with a substance abuse diagnosis typically included a 28-day hospitalization in a structured program that offered counseling, education, and an introduction to self-help groups. The case manager assigned upon admission coordinated the patient's acute treatment episode, serving as his or her primary therapist, advisor, and advocate. Upon discharge, the patient was referred to aftercare and assigned a second staff member or volunteer for continued counseling.

In the new reality, with patient care shifting to primarily outpatient therapies, formerly inpatient-only treatment centers have restructured their service delivery. Partial hospitalization and day-care programs have proliferated to replace long-term inpatient care management. Progressive programs offer a single case manager as care coordinator for managing patient care throughout the continuum. The assigned care coordinator adopts and monitors the patient for acute exacerbations, outpatient therapies, and required resource allocation and coordination. Over a course of therapy that may last weeks or months, the assigned case manager serves as the client's primary link with the program, providing individual counseling, group counseling, family counseling, education, and urine testing, as well as personal support and encouragement.

The case manager participates in a multidisciplinary process by presenting the patient at clinical case conferences, consulting with the medical or other service directors for medical or social management issues, and, finally, reporting patient progress to the utilization management team or payer organization.

• The Emerging Outpatient Case Management Concept

As mentioned previously, the escalating cost of treating substance abusers and chemical dependents has required development of new outpatient case management concepts to provide service to this special population. The concept that seems to be emerging emphasizes long-term patient treatment, intense patient–staff relationships, programmatic case management that builds on traditional alcohol and drug treatment models, and assistance with other human service concerns.

Emphasizing Long-Term Patient Relationships

Outpatient treatment for substance abusers is just as effective as inpatient treatment—and much less expensive. Longer outpatient stays are strongly correlated with more beneficial results.[1] The intensity and duration of treatment affects the quality of treatment outcomes. Recovery from substance abuse is a long-term process, and treatment is best provided in a program of at least one year's duration that establishes a long-term relationship between the patient and all program staff.[2]

Unfortunately, though, current reimbursement trends do not support long-term outpatient involvement. A recent report on health insurance plans for federal employees indicates that almost all health care plans impose a stringent limit on outpatient mental health and substance abuse treatment. Many existing insurer plans cover only 10 to 20 outpatient mental health visits, and coverage for substance abuse treatment is even less generous.[3]

Building on Traditional Alcohol Treatment Models

An emerging concept of case management—the one employed at Seton House—views case management as a complement to traditional alcohol and drug treatment services. With this philosophy in mind, the assigned case manager endeavors to improve the outpatient's status and postdischarge functioning and to bolster treatment effectiveness via outreach programs that enhance social stability through specific interventions. The case manager responds to the individualized needs of the client, links the client to needed services, functions as an advocate, and coordinates elements of the overall service delivery system.[4] The Enhanced Treatment through Induction and Case Management Project, a demonstration project funded by the National Institute of Drug Abuse, has as its goal the improvement of treatment retention and compliance as well as both short- and long-term treatment outcomes. In this vein, case management and patient advocacy strategies are expected to encourage substance abusers to remain in treatment and realize their treatment goals.[5]

Remembering Other Human Services

Traditional treatment programs can place too much emphasis on substance abuse as a primary condition warranting exclusive focus, sometimes ignoring other human service concerns, such as housing, jobs, and education, that directly affect a client's ability to engage in the treatment process. Nonresidential treatment for substance abusers requires the coordination of a variety of services, including detoxification, rehabilitation, relapse prevention, family treatment, HIV/AIDS education, vocational training, child-rearing classes, housing referrals, and more, depending on the needs of the individual.

Today's chemical dependents and substance abusers offer greater challenges to health care professionals than they did years ago. Patients addicted to cocaine or its derivative, crack, are more likely to suffer from complicated psychopathology and present with more complex medical problems than alcohol-only abusers. These patients are more difficult to engage in treatment, more likely to drop out of treatment, and relapse sooner than their alcohol-only counterparts.[6]

Similar to the mental health model for case management that evolved in response to deinstitutionalization, the enhanced substance abuse case management model is designed to assist a population of persons with multiple medical and social problems in making the transition from institutionalized care to independent living through outpatient-based or community service programs. As in the mental health model, the basic theory is that individual clients should utilize their own strengths and assets to acquire what they need—the case manager assisting them as "traveling companion and not travel agent."[7]

• Utilization Review and Cost Containment

A dramatic increase in volumes of chemically dependent clients combined with the rising cost of treatment has led to intensified managed care with increased emphasis on cost containment and accountability. Payer-based utilization management organizations provide experts to case manage chemical dependency clients. Case management of this type includes preadmission review of hospital stays, utilization review during treatment to assess the medical necessity of the services delivered, and contractual arrangements with preferred provider networks to direct the patient to the most cost-effective service provider.[8]

Although the treatment field is currently underfunded, some forecasters predict that managed care will improve the coordination of benefits. "Payers will establish mechanisms for coordinating all areas of benefits, especially those related to health, disability and worker's compensation. This will most likely be achieved utilizing case management models which integrate prevention, employee assistance and worksite medical and health network-based services."[9]

Several trends have emerged that may support the notion of enhanced outpatient case management. Because the point of entry into substance abuse treatment services usually is an outpatient source, such as a detoxification center or an emergency department, programmed services should be offered as a clinical model of service, not a hospital model of service. Programs also should demonstrate improved quality at reduced costs, because health reform and reimbursement initiatives will be based on clinical efficacy and outcomes. High-quality services and competitive pricing are the most likely strategies to achieve increased utilization and enhanced market share. Direct consumer marketing, formerly employed to attract paying patients, is less necessary in a managed care environment where fewer patients have the power to choose their provider of service. Chemical dependency programs will need to be structured, packaged, and negotiated with a new market in mind and new purchasers of care—for example, a self-insured company that wants an alcohol/drug/mental health care preferred provider organization, a health maintenance organization that wants to carve out alcohol/drug/mental health care, or a case management firm that is establishing a network of providers.

Professional licensing and certification standards have tightened for those involved in the delivery of direct services to privately insured substance abusers and chemical dependents. Current reimbursement and staffing patterns will need to be examined in order for an extended outpatient case management model to become widely operational in the private treatment field.

• Conclusion

Today's evolving and complex health care market commands restructured substance abuse and chemical dependency treatment programs that feature outpatient case management. Comprehensive case management should include care coordination across the care continuum, preferably led by a solitary case manager whose responsibilities include integration of the other human services so essential to this client group. In developing a program that effectively addresses the special needs of this chronically relapsing and noncompliant population, Seton House has found a way to secure the safe return of substance abusers and chemical dependents to their families, the work force, and the community.

References

1. Gerstein, D. R., and Harwood, H. J., editors. *Treating Drug Problems: A Study of the Evolution, Effectiveness, and Financing of Public and Private Drug Treatment Systems.* Washington, DC: National Academy Press, 1990.

2. Institute of Medicine. *Broadening the Base for Alcohol Treatment.* Washington, DC: National Academy Press, 1990.

3. Francis, W. Checkbook's guide to health insurance plans for federal employees. *Washington Consumers Checkbook Magazine,* 15th edition, pp. 43–44, Nov. 1992.

4. Patterson, D. Y. Rational rationing: the future of mental health care. Behavioral health care tomorrow: the rational dialogue conference on mental health practice in the era of managed care, (p. 11). Porta Valley, CA: Institute for Behavioral Healthcare, Sept. 1989.

5. Cole, P. A., Siegal, H. A., Forney, M. A., Rapp, R. C., Fisher, J. H., and Callejo, V. E. Jr. The enhanced treatment project. *Addiction & Recovery* 12(2):72–74, Mar.–Apr. 1992.

6. Wallace, J. Chemical dependence treatment for the '90s: promises and pitfalls. *EAPA Exchange* 20(4):2, 25, Apr. 1990.

7. Cole, p. 73.

8. Gray, B. H. *The Profit Motive and Patient Care: The Changing Accountability of Doctors and Hospitals.* Cambridge, MA: Harvard University Press, 1991.

9. Rodiguez, A. R. A vision of the behavioral healthcare industry. *Behavioral Healthcare Tomorrow* 1(1):16–18, Sept. 1992.

Chapter 19

Case Management Model: Rehabilitation

James A. Sliwa, DO

• Introduction

Rehabilitation strives to improve the functional status of individuals physically impaired or disabled by pain and to provide education for their families and caregivers. Employing a multidisciplinary team that includes physicians, nurses, psychologists, social workers, and physical, occupational, recreational, and speech therapists, the rehabilitation program replaces the traditional medical model of diagnosis and treatment with a model that assesses functional status and sets goals of treatment. However, because most practitioners in other fields of medicine know little about what can reasonably be accomplished during rehabilitation, patients' risk of becoming "lost in the system" may be greatest when they are referred for rehabilitation services. In this light, rehabilitation may represent the prototype of case management models.

The case management model used by the Rehabilitation Institute of Chicago helps patients achieve their maximum functional status and minimize secondary complications. The primary objectives of the model are threefold:

1. To make the referral for rehabilitation services at the appropriate time
2. To establish clear treatment goals and schedules for the rehabilitation team
3. To facilitate communication between the acute care and rehabilitation practitioners

In fulfilling these objectives, the case management program coordinates care and allocates resources in a timely and cost-effective manner.

This chapter describes the scope of rehabilitation services currently offered in the outpatient arena and highlights the case management model used by the Rehabilitation Institute of Chicago. It also discusses the importance of communication to development of an effective plan of care in terms of both financial benefits and functional improvement.

• Background and Scope of Practice

The past decade has seen explosive growth in rehabilitation services, particularly in outpatient programs. One recent hospital survey reports an increase in total outpatient visits from 778,000 to more than 2.2 million and a 76 percent increase in visits per rehabilitation facility over a nine-year period.[1] This growth has resulted in part from the wider spectrum of patients referred for rehabilitation services offered in diverse outpatient settings. Young victims of spinal cord trauma, workers suffering lower back injuries, and the elderly with declining functional status are all being referred for outpatient rehabilitation services, which can now be provided in freestanding rehabilitation therapy centers, acute care hospitals with or without rehabilitation units, and the private practice offices of physiatrists and therapists.

The scope of rehabilitation service offerings is as variable and as broad as the scope of providers. For example, a hospital without an outpatient rehabilitation unit may offer only individual services such as physical therapy, concentrating on the short-term treatment of impairments such as outpatient gait training or joint mobilization after orthopedic surgery. Many outpatient programs today focus on specific disabilities such as head injury, stroke, pulmonary rehabilitation, back pain, or chronic pain management. Freestanding rehabilitation hospitals or community hospitals with rehabilitation units are more likely to provide a full range of services comparable to the comprehensive rehabilitation services they offer on an inpatient basis. In addition to rehabilitation services provided by physicians and nurses, these freestanding facilities offer the following:

- Occupational therapy
- Physical therapy
- Psychology
- Speech–language pathology
- Orthotics
- Prosthetics
- Therapeutic recreation
- Social work
- Vocational rehabilitation
- Rehabilitation engineering

In general, neurologists, neurosurgeons, internists, and orthopedic surgeons are the major referral sources for rehabilitation services, but development of outpatient services is largely determined by the practice type of referring physicians and the range of disabilities seen on the inpatient rehabilitation unit. For example, a community hospital that provides inpatient rehabilitation care for predominantly stroke and amputee victims will certainly require different outpatient services than will a large freestanding rehabilitation hospital that provides inpatient care for more specialized disabilities such as spinal cord injury, traumatic brain injury, or burns. Likewise, a community hospital with a large and active orthopedic group treating back and spinal disorders will find it necessary to provide back rehabilitation, pain management services, and work-hardening programs.

• The Program Model

This section describes the case management model used by the Rehabilitation Institute of Chicago to achieve its care objectives. It discusses the collaboration between physician and insurance case manager in devising a patient care plan, the appropriateness of inpatient versus outpatient care, and the factors that help determine the course and duration of treatment.

Key Participants

Outpatient case management at the Rehabilitation Institute of Chicago is a team effort. The attending physician, a specialist in rehabilitative and physical medicine, coordinates the patient's entire course of treatment. Clinically speaking, then, the rehabilitation physician is the true case manager. But the patient's insurance company assigns its own case manager to ensure that the Institute provides only the services the patient needs, in the most cost-effective manner possible. The insurance company's case manager keeps abreast of the patient's progress through an appointed staff liaison—a social worker or nurse therapist from the patient's care-giving team. Upon the patient's referral to the Institute, the physician and the insurance case manager together assess his or her needs and establish an individualized, coordinated care plan and treatment regime.

Inpatient versus Outpatient Care

With few exceptions, outpatient rehabilitation treatments are less intensive than inpatient treatments. Although a minimum of three hours of daily therapy is the standard for inpatient rehabilitation, the typical outpatient treatment program entails one to three hours of therapy, one to three days per week. Outpatient pain management and work-hardening programs are notable exceptions to the rule, providing daily treatment and either a full day of treatment or a gradual increase to that level.

Besides a lower intensity of required care, outpatient treatment might be appropriate when a narrower scope of services is needed. Inpatient rehabilitation provides daily physician supervision, rehabilitation nursing, psychological support, social work, therapeutic recreational services, and physical, occupational, and speech therapy. Rehabilitation outpatients may require one or two of these services but normally not the full range.

Course and Duration of Treatment

Although the needs, focus, and length of treatment will vary depending on diagnosis, one important distinction for the case management team is the progressive versus nonprogressive causes of impairment. For example, an individual rendered paraplegic by trauma may be left with a fixed, unchanging deficit, whereas an individual with paraplegia as a result of multiple sclerosis may experience unpredictable, progressive changes in functional status. Although the case management objectives for the two cases might be the same, the plans of care would be quite different.

There is no average duration of treatment for outpatient rehabilitation. The severity and nature of the disability, medical complications, coexisting medical conditions, cognitive status, and motivation all influence the progress, duration, and outcome of treatment. A young, healthy individual may easily complete a course of treatment for mechanical low back pain in four to six weeks, whereas an older individual with multiple medical problems and a traumatic brain injury may make slow but steady progress for months. The rule of thumb for outpatient rehabilitation is to continue treatment as long as the patient is progressing toward documentable and reasonable goals, such as decreased pain or improved functional status.

• The Need for Open Communication

No matter what the nature of the impairment, the key to a successful rehabilitation care plan is communication among all members of the care-giving team. In rehabilitation, unlike many other medical specialties, treatment is dispersed among a number of practitioners, sometimes in a variety of settings, and most rehabilitation outpatients continue to receive treatment from one or more acute care physicians as well. Communication, both among members of the rehabilitation team and between the acute care and rehabilitation practitioners, is essential to helping the patient accomplish maximum function in a timely, cost-effective manner.

Responsibility for keeping these lines of communication open rests with the insurance company's case manager. The insurance case manager follows a patient's ongoing tests, medical treatments, and therapies in addition to all the input and orders from attending or consulting physicians. Contacting the rehabilitation physician will quickly confirm whether the patient is indeed an appropriate candidate for participation in a rehabilitation program, is participating in therapy, and is progressing toward established goals.

More challenging is facilitating communication between acute care and rehabilitative practitioners. This can be a major issue when additional testing, treatment, or a deteriorating medical condition interferes with therapy or results in a decline in functional status. For example, a worker with emphysema who is injured on the job and undergoing rehabilitation for a back injury may not be able to participate effectively in therapy if the emphysema flares up. Therapy may have to be postponed until the medical condition improves, and it is up to the insurance case manager first to determine when therapy may be resumed and then to arrange the continuing rehabilitation care plan.

By acting as liaison between acute and rehabilitative care, facilitating interdisciplinary communication, and directing patients to the appropriate physicians when questions or problems arise, the insurance case manager minimizes conflicts among health care providers and delineates the boundaries of treatment for each discipline.

• Program Benefits

The financial benefits of providing effective case management for rehabilitation patients will depend on whether care is delivered in a rehabilitation hospital or on an outpatient basis, and on the intensity of treatment, the number and types of treatments required, the convenience of the facility's location, the required duration of service, and the need for ancillary services. Surely the savings offered by outpatient versus inpatient rehabilitation service delivery are apparent. Less intensive therapies, no room charges, and less need for physician supervision make outpatient rehabilitation the cost-efficient choice for many patient types.

In the final analysis, however, rehabilitation will be thought of not in terms of cost savings but, rather, in terms of improved functional status and quality of life. The financial benefits of rehabilitation may be difficult to document, but improvements in the function and quality of a patient's life are easily visible and greatly rewarding. Together, the patient, physician, and insurance case manager can best determine the true value of ongoing rehabilitation and the real benefits of treatment.

• Conclusion

In recent years, outpatient rehabilitation services have experienced phenomenal growth. The scope of services is diverse, ranging from a focus on specific disabilities to provision of a full range of services comparable to that offered on an inpatient basis. Effective coordination of such rehabilitation services depends on successful implementation of a case management program characterized by team work and open communication. A program such as the model used by the Rehabilitation Institute of Chicago can be instrumental in improving patients' quality of life and can speed

their functional return to society following a disabling injury or event—
and that is a service to everyone.

Reference

1. Sliwa, J. A., editor. *Outpatient Rehabilitation Services: A Guide to Planning and Management.* Chicago: American Hospital Publishing, 1991.

Chapter 20

Case Management Model: Oncology

Eileen Smyth Groh, Dorothy A. Calabrese, and Mary Lynn Droughton

• Introduction

Oncology is among the fastest-growing outpatient therapeutics. New outpatient oncology programs are proliferating with the wider availability of advanced technologies and pharmaceuticals and home infusion programs. Screening procedures and early intervention with innovative therapies are allowing greater numbers of cancer patients to effect a cure or to live longer, more productive lives. In the next decade, more than 90 percent of cancer care will be delivered in ambulatory settings and physicians' offices.

Because, as a disease process, cancer threatens to overtake heart disease as the number one cause of morbidity and mortality by the year 2000, establishing more cancer care programs in all kinds of settings seems a logical direction to take. The practice of oncology will see more multidisciplinary teams of caregivers providing patients with a wide range of services, from diagnosis through comprehensive cancer therapies. For example, holistic cancer care will offer services such as pain control, hospice, patient and family grieving and support, and respite care, in addition to therapeutics. Inpatient oncology services will likely be limited to initial therapeutic intervention, experimental treatments requiring pharmacokinetics, and to patients requiring major surgery as the preferred intervention. Patient support and case management will follow the entire continuum — from initial screening and diagnosis to tertiary-level therapies.[1]

In terms of case management, purchasers of services are looking for programs that provide high-quality care, a customer orientation, and a full array of services with convenient one-stop shopping. For cancer patients, such a program is essential. However, oncology case management involves a wide spectrum of diseases, and its therapeutics incorporate diverse medical specialties and professional disciplines and a host of support services. Assisting patients and their families through a long and often arduous course of treatment requires a high level of communication between disciplines and services.

The Cleveland Clinic Foundation, a tertiary care center encompassing a 1,000-bed hospital and an extensive outpatient clinic complex, has established separate case management models for specific oncology patient populations. This chapter presents three models—medical oncology, head and neck oncology, and urologic oncology—that illustrate the challenges and potential benefits of oncology case management.

• Model 1. Medical Oncology

The Hematology and Medical Oncology Outpatient Clinic at the Cleveland Clinic Foundation serves the patients of 16 medical staff and 9 fellows, handling approximately 35,000 visits per year. The clinic is staffed by five full-time registered nurses (RNs) and two nursing unit assistants. In addition, there are five nurse clinicians (RNs with advanced specialty training) in dedicated positions serving specific clinical and research programs. The outpatient chemotherapy treatment area, located conveniently adjacent to the outpatient clinic, administers approximately 8,800 treatments per year and is staffed by eight full-time RNs specializing in chemotherapy administration and one nursing unit assistant.

A clinical nurse specialist (CNS) (a master's-prepared RN) manages both the outpatient clinic and the chemotherapy treatment area. In this collaborative, cooperative model, case management responsibilities essentially are shared by the entire care-giving team.

Care Management in the Outpatient Setting

Continued alterations in patterns of hospital reimbursement, especially diagnosis-related groups (DRGs), have created new incentives to provide more services in the outpatient setting. Although most medical oncology outpatients come to the clinic for routine physician visits, the clinic nursing staff also perform a number of elective or urgent procedures traditionally rendered only in inpatient settings.

Orders for patient diagnostics, therapeutics, and support services at the clinic are initiated by the physician. For patients with a previously established treatment plan, the clinic nurses' responsibilities include assessing the patient on each visit, carrying out the plan of care, and notifying the physician of significant findings. Other essential patient services, such as lab work, routine transfusion, hydration, IV electrolytes, antiemetics, and so on, are scheduled as needed.

Life-threatening situations are referred to the hospital emergency department (ED), although stable patients requiring urgent care are instructed to report to the outpatient clinic area. Most emergent and urgent visits originate with a patient call to an oncology nurse clinician, a staff medical oncologist, or a fellow, who in turn calls the outpatient nurse with an assessment of the patient's condition and initial orders. The outpatient clinic nurse and nurse clinician or physician perform additional assessment on arrival and collaborate on a plan of care.

Although this plan typically may involve up to eight hours of assessment, intervention, and reevaluation by the outpatient nurse, other support services may be required and normally are on-call to the clinic area. For example, a social worker is available for counseling, assistance with social and financial issues, and home care arrangements. A respiratory therapist, a dietitian, and a skin care specialist are available for further assessment and intervention as indicated. And nurse clinicians or CNSs from other areas such as otolaryngology, urology, neurology, and neurosurgery are available for one-to-one consultation if required.

Establishment of the Care Continuum

Should an outpatient's condition warrant admission, the CNS, the nurse clinician, or the physician initiates the plan for acute care and the clinic nurse facilitates the patient's admission. This process establishes the patient care continuum and potentially reduces length of stay. For example, a patient being admitted for suspected neutropenic sepsis will have baseline lab work drawn as well as blood, urine, and sputum cultures. Intravenous fluids and IV antibiotics are started in the clinic. A nursing report is called in to the receiving hospital staff nurse and the patient is transported directly to the hospital nursing unit.

Similarly, patients being discharged from the hospital are referred back to the clinic for follow-up care. When chemotherapy regimens require hospitalization, appropriate lab work is completed and chemotherapy initiated in the outpatient chemotherapy treatment area to facilitate the admission process and limit length of stay. Each of these procedures enhances the continuum of care for individual patients.

• Model 2. Head and Neck Oncology

The head and neck oncology program comprises a complex, high-cost, high-risk patient population utilizing multiple resources. These patients often present multiple medical problems — for example, chronic obstructive pulmonary disease (COPD), alcoholism, malnutrition — and require additional levels of service or care. The head and neck oncology patient may require nursing care related to airway management, deglutition, nutrition, mouth and wound care, pain management, and communication. More pronounced psychosocial issues, including coping with alterations in communication, disfigurement, alcoholism, codependency, cognitive deficits, and finances, make this patient population especially challenging. Thus, it is essential to provide a well-organized and flexible plan of care to meet the special and diverse physical and psychosocial needs of this client population.

The Clinical Nurse Specialist as Case Manager

The Cleveland Clinic Foundation's head and neck oncology case management model is designed to provide a continuum of care throughout the patient's episode of illness, whatever the setting. The model employs an interdisciplinary group practice in which the CNS is the ultimate case manager and clinical coordinator for both inpatient and outpatient care.

The CNS is supported by an inpatient case manager (ICM) and an outpatient case manager (OCM) assigned responsibility for patient care/coordination in their respective settings. The CNS oversees the patient care administered by both the ICM and the OCM to ensure a continuum of care. Head and neck oncology patients who require surgery as a part of their treatment plan are initially seen by the outpatient case manager. The OCM coordinates all preoperative testing and consults (for example, social work, dentistry, speech pathology) and performs nursing assessments and educational sessions regarding the preoperative and postoperative courses of treatment, nursing care, case management, discharge needs, and related self-care.

Preservation of the Care Continuum

By having the same team of case managers follow the entire care plan — beginning before hospital admission, through the acute phase, and after discharge and referral back to the outpatient clinic — the head and neck oncology case management program achieves a true continuum of care. Team members thus have an active and ongoing role in providing seamless patient care.

Surgery patients are not admitted prior to their procedures but, instead, arrive the morning of surgery and are admitted afterward. As the patient's scheduled surgery approaches, the OCM communicates the outpatient nursing assessments, interventions, and evaluations to the ICM and the CNS. The inpatient case manager assumes responsibility during the patient's hospitalization. Prior to discharge, the patient/family and all three case managers review the discharge plan and the patient's requirements for aftercare. Head and neck surgery patients are commonly discharged with tracheostomies, enteral feeding needs, wounds, drains, pain, and altered communication; patients and families must learn how to provide appropriate care.

Between 24 and 48 hours after discharge, the ICM calls the patient to evaluate the patient or family's ability to perform self-care and revises the plan if necessary. The ICM communicates this evaluation to the OCM, who then continues to monitor and revise the care plan according to the patient's status. Patient progress is monitored through home care nurses and frequent clinic visits.

Evolution of the Case Management Model

Before implementing the head and neck oncology case management model at Cleveland Clinic Foundation, the director of medical/surgical nursing, the nurse manager of the otolaryngology unit, a charge nurse from the outpatient otolaryngology clinic, and the CNS met to design a case management pilot for the head and neck patient population. The pilot program was designed to manage the care of three case types: total laryngectomies, partial laryngectomies, and neck dissections (at that time DRG 49). Using retrospective chart reviews, the committee designed coordinated care tracks that included not only physician and nursing assessments and care but also actions, where appropriate, by a social worker, a dietitian, a respiratory therapist, a home care nurse, a dentist, and a speech pathologist. The committee also designed pilot goals, case manager job descriptions, and an overall implementation plan. The CNS was to function in both outpatient and inpatient areas.

Once the foundation for case management was laid, two otolaryngologists agreed to pilot the model with their patients and provided their input regarding the overall case management project. Once their support was secured, the pilot committee discussed the model with other members of the multidisciplinary head and neck oncology team and with staff nurses in both inpatient and outpatient areas. The physicians' and nurses' recommendations and revisions were incorporated into the model. Interested nurses with special expertise were interviewed for case manager positions, and two were selected and oriented by the CNS.

Program Benefits

The initial goals of the pilot program were to reduce length of stay, decrease the number of hospital readmissions, contain costs, and provide high-quality care throughout the patient's episode of illness. The following data were collected during the one-year period beginning September 1, 1990, and ending August 1, 1991.

The mix of the three case types in the pilot program involved 45 patients. Following are the case types and the number of patients in each:

- Total laryngectomy (11 patients)
- Partial laryngectomy (6 patients)
- Neck dissections (28 patients)

The total and partial laryngectomy and neck dissection patients (DRG 49) were allowed a 7.4-day hospitalization. On October 1, 1991, change ensued, with partial and total laryngectomies assigned the new DRG 482 (tracheostomy with mouth, larynx, or pharynx disorder) and allotted a stay of 14.2 days. Neck dissections remained DRG 49 and were allotted 7.4 days. Tables 20-1 and 20-2 show the continuing decline in length of stay from the inception of the head and neck pilot program and following the introduction of DRG 482. Outliers were most frequently attributed to complicated medical diagnoses (for example, oropharyngeal cutaneous fistulas, high drain output, aspiration pneumonia, deep-vein thrombosis), awaiting extended care

Table 20-1.   Actual Lengths of Stay (LOS) for DRG 49 during the Head and Neck Pilot Program (Sept. 1, 1990–Aug. 1, 1991)

Case Types	DRG LOS	Actual LOS	Number of Patients
Partial Laryngectomies	7.4 Days	6 Days	3
(DRG 49)		8–15 Days	3
		Total:	6
Total Laryngectomies	7.4 Days	8–12 Days	9
(DRG 49)		22 Days	2
		Total:	11
Neck Dissections	7.4 Days	2 Days	2
(DRG 49)		3 Days	1
		4 Days	5
		5 Days	7
		6 Days	2
		7 Days	2
		9–18 Days	8
		5 Months	1
		Total:	28

Table 20-2.   Average Lengths of Stay (ALOS) in the Head and Neck Program Following the Introduction of DRG 482 (Jan. 1–Sept. 30, 1992)

DRG	January–March	April–June	July–September
	Number of Patients/ALOS	Number of Patients/ALOS	Number of Patients/ALOS
49 (Allotted LOS 7.4)	10/7.1	12/6.6	8/4.9
482 (Allotted LOS 14.2)	32/8.8	28/8.9	28/8.5

facility placement, and family unwillingness to assume care responsibilities. Once discharged from the acute care setting, these patients often required continuing nursing care.

Through constant contact with patients at home and in nursing facilities, the OCM was able to identify patient problems early and address them in the outpatient setting, preventing hospital readmissions. Examples of early interventions include placement of nasogastric tubes, coordination of resources, patient teaching of wound care, and enteral feeding. Follow-up self-care and reinforcement teaching responsibilities were assumed by the home care nurse, which allowed the patient to be managed at home with family support systems and without compromising the quality or continuity of care.

• Model 3. Urologic Oncology

Case management of the urologic oncology population is a relatively new concept. The goal is to provide high-quality, cost-effective medical and nursing care through a coordinated, interdisciplinary approach that affords continuity for both inpatients and outpatients.

At Cleveland Clinic Foundation, the urologic oncology case management model is comparable to the head and neck model. A CNS for urologic/oncology acts as clinical coordinator for both inpatient and outpatient settings. In the urology program, an inpatient nursing case manager oversees the acute care phase and coordinates the care required for needs identified during hospitalization and following discharge. The physical and psychosocial needs of these patients usually are not as complex as those of patients in the head and neck program.

Patient Types Managed in the Outpatient Setting

Case management is applied primarily to two groups of urologic oncology patients in the outpatient setting. The first group includes patients who are surgical candidates: patients with kidney cancer (requiring radical or partial nephrectomy), patients with prostate cancer (requiring radical prostatectomy), and patients with bladder cancer (requiring cystectomy with urinary diversion). The second group includes patients with advanced prostate cancer whose disease is managed with hormone therapy.

Surgical Candidates

Preoperative teaching for surgical candidates is accomplished by the CNS or the nurses in the outpatient setting. Written instructions regarding major surgical procedures are mailed to patients several weeks before their scheduled surgery. During the presurgical assessment visit, the CNS answers the patient's questions and discusses the surgery and probable hospital care and after-care, including pain management, respiratory care, and activities of daily living. After this assessment, the potential needs of both patient and family are identified and communicated to the inpatient case manager.

Following admission to the hospital, surgical patients are placed on a coordinated care track (CCT), which serves as a guideline for care during hospitalization. Variation from the intended CCT is evaluated by the nurse case manager (NCM) to assess the appropriateness of or need for modified nursing intervention. Keeping in mind the medical and nursing goal to pro-vide cost-efficient, high-quality patient care, the CCT can be modified according to patient need. Table 20-3 illustrates the benefits of the CCT in terms of declining length of stay for radical prostatectomy patients.

Weekly interdisciplinary discharge rounds identify inpatient, discharge, and outpatient care needs. Ongoing communication and input from social work, home care, the NCM, the staff nurse, and the CNS facilitate early identification of patient needs. Early interventions for both the acute and the discharge planning phases can then be implemented.

As case manager, the NCM's primary responsibilities are assessment and reevaluation. Following discharge, the NCM evaluates patient progress with a follow-up call. Should a problem be identified during this call, a return visit or other appropriate referral will be scheduled. Patients may call the CNS or NCM at any time to discuss problems or concerns. This is a valu-able mechanism, because it enables the case manager and the CNS to iden-tify problems before they require medical intervention.

For example, a patient who resides nearby and experiences postopera-tive drainage from a surgical incision would come to the outpatient area for evaluation by the CNS. If the patient lives at a distance, a visiting nurse would be sent to his or her home to assess the wound. These types of inter-ventions often prevent costly visits to the ED.

Table 20-3. ALOS for Radical Prostatectomy Patients on the Coordinated Care Track (Apr. 1–Dec. 31, 1992)

DRG	April–June Number of Patients/ALOS	July–September Number of Patients/ALOS	October–December Number of Patients/ALOS
334	5.0/7.4 (HCFA LOS 8.9)	6/7.83 (HCFA LOS 8.9)	15/6.80 (HCFA LOS 8.2)
335	16/6.62 (HCFA LOS 7.4)	16/6.29 (HCFA LOS 7.4)	11/5.47 (HCFA LOS 6.9)

HCFA = Health Care Financing Administration.

Advanced Prostate Cancer Patients

The second group of urologic oncology patients managed in the outpatient setting are those with metastatic prostate cancer managed by monthly hormone injections (leuprolide or goserelin acetate). These patients are seen monthly in a nurse-managed clinic. The clinic's primary purpose is to offer standardized routine patient assessment and to identify potential problems. The nursing staff in this area practice within certain protocols regarding blood work and scheduled physician appointments. As a result of the strong educational component of the program, which is taught by nurses, these patients are particularly astute regarding their medical condition and potential complications.

The metastatic prostate cancer program has proven quite effective. For example, several patients with impending spinal cord compression were identified by nursing staff during outpatient visits. The nurses' assessment and subsequent early medical intervention prevented serious complications for these patients.

• Financial Implications of Nurse-Administered Case Management Programs

The financial success of an outpatient case management program will depend on controlling the following elements:

- Cost per case
- Resource utilization
- Admission/readmission rates
- Professional/technical reimbursement

Gaining control of costs should be considered a by-product of a high-quality program, and a nurse-run case management program embraces the quality philosophy. The nurse case manager is in a unique position to assess, plan, and evaluate the dimensions of care for his or her caseload. Patients' needs are thereby defined and strategies implemented with close attention given to the quality, appropriateness, and cost of care. The care continuum is maintained across inpatient and outpatient arenas, and unnecessary admissions and costly complications are thus avoided or subject to early identification and intervention.

Carefully managing resources, including supplies, durable medical equipment, home care services, and the number of physician and nurse visits, is the most efficient way to control cost per case. Case management has provided the level of aggregate analysis to predict what resources will be necessary to achieve positive clinical outcomes in specific patient populations. This has been accomplished through a continuous quality improvement (CQI) process aimed at changing or enhancing practice. Case managers monitor patient progress and outcomes and, in turn, identify problems or opportunities for restructuring care for the benefit of their patients.

Hospital readmissions are a costly venture for providers and for patients and their families. Under the current system, most hospital readmissions are denied reimbursement if they occur within 30 days of discharge. The case manager in the outpatient arena has the unique opportunity to avoid readmissions by performing assessments and adjusting care intervention and resource allocation as the patient's condition and events change. For example, the CNS case manager in the head and neck program at Cleveland Clinic Foundation has been able to recommend skilled care visits to manage increasing problems with complex dressings, change dietary supplements to combat declining weight, and increase the frequency of clinic visits to detect and prevent potential complications, such as drug interaction, persistent pain, or skin problems.

By providing such depth of service and the supporting documentation, the case managers also have proven effective in optimizing reimbursement for both physician and institution. Many third-party payers are reluctant to provide payment if procedures or visits are not clearly documented in detail. With qualified nurse clinicians and clinical nurse specialists dedicated to the tasks of evaluating aggregate data, monitoring patient care, and educating other team members, oncology case management provides high-quality care with all the documentation that patients, practitioners, providers, and payers require.

• Conclusion

Oncology case management at Cleveland Clinic Foundation has been a great asset for all concerned. Because serving the diverse clinical and psychosocial needs of cancer patients demands careful coordination by an interdisciplinary team, highly organized case management is integral to high-quality patient care and cost-effectiveness. Case management provides the continuity of care needed by this patient population.

Reference

1. American Hospital Association. *Meditrends, 1991.* Chicago: AHA, 1991.

Chapter 21

Case Management Model: Cardiovascular Services

Mary Ann House-Fancher

• Introduction

The cardiovascular center (CVC) at Shands Hospital, in Gainesville, Florida, has a pilot approach to case management for the cardiovascular outpatient. Shands Hospital is a nonprofit institution affiliated with the University of Florida Health Science Center. The program's primary purpose is to provide efficient and effective medical and nursing care to clients who present with potential or actual alterations in cardiovascular function. The case management goals of the outpatient CVC are as follows:

- To promptly assess individual patients presenting or referred for services
- To identify specific client needs through timely triage and appropriate referrals for care
- To make referrals for extended or further medical evaluation
- To develop a specific plan of care that implements a therapeutic regime and then evaluates and documents the client's response

By providing expeditious patient management, diagnostic procedural scheduling, quality monitoring, and data collection, the Shands CVC daily fulfills its case management goals and successfully coordinates outpatient services for referral patients whose care might otherwise be difficult to organize or require hospital admission. This chapter examines the Shands model and describes its success.

• New Program Development

The Shands cardiovascular outpatient case management model was spawned by needs and deficiencies identified in cardiovascular care, by discussions with the directors of inpatient cardiovascular services, and by a comprehensive analysis of the hospital's programs, mission, and goals for the future. Because both the university and the hospital had pursued client-centered care for the inpatient sector, they naturally supported development of similar models in the outpatient arena.

The clinic's outpatients are primarily referrals from other medical outreach programs and physicians in the county, state, and outlying regions. As a university-based program with medical and nursing schools, Shands offers these patients diagnostic or therapeutic procedures not available in their residential community hospitals. For example, many such patients are referred to the hospital's heart transplant program or for experimental drug protocols and treatment modalities. Others are same-day cardiology or cardiovascular surgery clients. To meet the functional challenges posed by a growing subacute population, Shands has implemented a program that predefines patient care outcomes, time frames, and critical pathways over the entire continuum of patient care.

A significant number of end-stage congestive heart failure clients are admitted to the hospital for repeated procedures and medications. The new CVC's infusion and procedure rooms provide outpatients with intravenous drugs, cardiac and pulmonary assessment, and advanced hemodynamic monitoring. Instead of being admitted as inpatients, clients are now treated for six to eight hours with advanced drug therapy, assessed by a case manager or nurse practitioner, and discharged home at the end of the treatment regimen.

• The Case Manager's Roles and Functions

The focus of the Shands CVC is to provide comprehensive, client-centered care, while monitoring critical pathways and providing clinical education and leadership to the staff. Because the chief intent of the cardiovascular case management model is to facilitate rapid entry into the CVC, but with thorough clinical evaluation and assessment, each patient is assigned to a clinician with advanced experience and skill in cardiovascular nursing. These advanced nurse practitioners fulfill the core responsibilities of outpatient case management: patient triage and management, patient education, and program evaluation.

As case manager, the advanced nurse practitioner arranges the client's clinical assessment, assists in scheduling, and monitors patient progress. His or her advanced knowledge, ready availability, and leadership form a strong foundation for the program. The case manager improves client care by:

- Collaborating with the primary staff in establishing and evaluating the medical/nursing component of the client's critical pathway
- Collaborating with other health professionals to establish and integrate the client's care and to evaluate the overall critical pathway

- Providing independent advanced assessment of all clients
- Acting as clinical advisor to the nursing staff for changes in client acuity

With such close and expert guidance, patients are piloted through what might otherwise be a complex maze of cross-referrals and unnecessary or duplicative diagnostic tests.

At the CVC, the triage and same-day service allow clients and referring centers to plan a schedule that more appropriately serves clients' clinical needs and conditions. With a certified nurse practitioner with advanced skill in cardiovascular nursing as primary case manager, clients are assessed, triaged, and referred appropriately to subspecialists. Any laboratory, radiology, or cardiovascular testing required is ordered, completed, and available on the unit when the attending specialist consults with the patient. Early, coordinated test ordering avoids the potential abuse or overutilization of laboratory and other ancillary procedures. Patient workups are completed efficiently and rapidly according to predefined critical pathways aligned with the client's diagnosis, clinical condition, and unique medical and social needs. Because many CVC patients are elderly or medically compromised, the case manager serves an especially valuable function for these patients in minimizing the trauma and frustration of a prolonged visit.

A care delivery model coordinated and supervised by expert clinicians has one distinct advantage in the outpatient setting: With their expertise and experience, nurse practitioners can intervene and alter care pathways beyond the strict pathway overseen by managers with less expertise. Thus, these advanced clinician managers may have a substantial positive impact on quality of care, client outcomes, and resource utilization. At present, there are no studies to compare traditional pathway models to units that incorporate case management by advanced clinicians. Such studies are certainly warranted, and might well fuel the proliferation of this model.

The cardiovascular center staff were at first frustrated by their inability to properly educate the many clients and families they saw daily. Conflicting time commitments, work loads, and the complexity of the client population made the education effort nearly impossible. However, because advanced clinicians already had the expertise to educate clients, families, and staff, the case manager role soon expanded to include such services. Now, formal client and family classes, a variety of written materials, point-of-service education for individual clients, and bedside teaching are all part of the model.

Another responsibility of the nurse case manager is to collect data related to the utilization of the laboratory and ancillary testing procedures, and data on patient outcomes. Because the advanced nurse practitioner follows each client in the outpatient cardiology service, clinical assessments and resource utilization are easily monitored and documented, as are client variances and responses to therapy. To quantify the impact of the advanced nurse practitioner case management model, measurable targets were established for these data. These included:

- Time of referral to client appointment (to reduce waiting time for patients and referring physicians)
- Resources expended, for example, in laboratory and heart station utilization (to reduce repeat studies, gather data from the patient's history and previous testing, and eliminate duplication of unnecessary data)
- Number of clients seen in the infusion or procedure room (to increase the number of patients seen and reduce hospital admissions)
- Time to complete history/physical and client workup for designated outcomes, such as cardiac catheterization, surgery consult, interventional procedures (to reduce the waiting time for patients scheduled for outpatient or same-day admit procedures)
- Client, family, physician, and nurse satisfaction reports (to increase satisfaction of not only patients and families but also physicians and nurses)
- Staff retention in the CVC area

• Program Benefits

Financial and quality management incentives are paramount to the success of a cardiovascular outpatient case management model. Same-day service and prescheduled, coordinated appointments for new clients and referrals enhance patient flow through the system. In a traditional setting with attending physicians, fellows, and resident training programs, it could take three to four weeks for a client to be admitted and actually evaluated by an attending physician.

This pilot model, featuring advanced nurse practitioners as case managers, has indeed produced marked benefits for patients, staff, administrators, and payers alike. Patients are better satisfied with their treatment outcomes, staff are delighted with improved patient compliance, and administrators and payers marvel at the reduction in resources expended. By eliminating admission to the hospital, expediting patient access and flow through the system, and reducing overutilization of laboratory and diagnostic procedures, excessive cost factors are eliminated. And every client enjoys an uninterrupted continuum of care from inpatient to outpatient areas, guided by a holistic plan of care designed for his or her specific clinical and psychosocial needs.

• Conclusion

At a time when innovative delivery systems are required to meet the needs of a changing health care system, development of a client-centered outpatient case management model is fundamental. But establishing a truly effective outpatient case management program that encompasses preadmission testing and comprehensive outpatient diagnostic and therapeutic services for cardiovascular clients can be a trying process.

Shands Hospital's successful plan for implementation included objectives to ensure rapid access to the system, a swift but thorough clinical assessment, and — above all — safe, coordinated, and efficacious patient care management. As case managers, advanced nurse clinicians with cardiovascular experience lend the program their broad knowledge base, expertise, and versatility in meeting individual patient needs, ensuring a continuum of care, and promoting better client outcomes.

In short, the outpatient case management model for cardiovascular care has streamlined the allocation of resources, contained costs, and improved patient satisfaction at Shands Hospital. As the general population ages, health reform efforts will intensify, and new payment mechanisms will mold new care delivery systems. Organized clinical case management models that can achieve these goals will reign supreme.

Bibliography

Ahrens, T. S. Nurse clinician model of managed care. *AACN Clinical Issues in Critical Care Nursing* 3(4):761–68, 1992.

Ahrens, T. S., and Padwojski, A. Economic impact of advanced clinicians. *Nursing Management* 19(6):64D–F, June 1988.

Goodnough, S., Bines, A., and Schneider, W. The effect of clinical expertise on patient outcome. *Critical Care Medicine* 14(4):358, Apr. 1986.

Zander, K. Managed care within acute care settings: design and implementation via nursing case management. *Health Care Supervisor* 6(2):27–43, Jan. 1988.

Chapter 22

Case Management Model: Ambulatory Surgery

Mary Jo Breslin

• Introduction

The past decade has seen phenomenal growth in outpatient surgical procedures and a proliferation of hospital-based and freestanding ambulatory surgical facilities. Surgeons have become more subspecialized within their individual service specialties, discovering safer and more effective procedures to achieve minimally invasive surgical intervention.[1] This evolution, fostered by advanced technologies, new pharmaceuticals, and payer mandates, has conferred novel stature to the ambulatory surgical arena. Procedures formerly requiring four- to seven-day hospital stays have become same-day or short-stay procedures. While these procedures ultimately result in reduced length of stay, they also offer care management challenges for accommodating higher patient volumes and new patient types undergoing more intensive procedures.

By now, most organizations are revamping established programs to assist patients through a complex outpatient processing system. The primary objective of these programs is to provide convenient access and safe discharge following newly approved, minimally invasive surgical procedures. Short-stay observation and aftercare considerations for patients discharged directly to their homes or communities have required patients, providers, physicians, and payers to change the way they address the healing and recovery process.

This chapter looks at the need for ambulatory surgery case management programs and discusses the role of care mapping as a component of their implementation. It also describes issues such as financial incentives, the impact of the case management model on medical management, and recent trends in ambulatory care.

• The Need for Case Management

As a result of industry trends, providers and practitioners are organizing more comprehensive programs to accommodate this changing environment.

The need for special emphasis on patient convenience and safety, quality of care, system efficiencies, cost control, and coordinated resource allocation across the care continuum is paramount to new ambulatory program development. Further and particularly as a result of the physician reimbursement decline under a resource-based relative value scale (RBRVS) payment system, physician convenience, scheduling, and practice efficiencies are also in order.

Traditionally, the physician scheduled the patient for a surgical procedure and advised the patient to contact the hospital for more specific arrangements. However, because of stricter payer mandates and more stringent preoperative processing requirements, today's system is more complex for the physician, the physician's office staff, and the patient. Navigating the system and the admission process usually is the responsibility of the patient and family. Some hospitals no longer have as much control in orchestrating ambulatory patient flow and problem solving, often restricted by resource availability, inadequate processing systems, commingled services, and the brevity of patient encounters.

Overall, both freestanding and hospital-based facilities face varied and multiple challenges in programmatic service delivery. Several of these distinctions are outlined in figure 22-1, which enumerates advantages and disadvantages of these program types. However unique these different programs are, a comprehensive patient care management system must be in place. Existence of a focused case management program facilitates the processing of the various components of care as well as safe, efficient, high-quality care delivery for the surgical outpatient.

To achieve optimal patient outcomes within a limited time frame, ambulatory surgical care must be closely and comprehensively managed. The program must consistently meet the diverse needs of patients, payers, and physicians as well as achieve objectives and cost controls established by the organization or governing body. These are best illustrated by recent initiatives of physician–hospital organizations (PHOs) to package prices for negotiating service fees with managed care or local business contractors. Thus, organized case management programs offer untold value and play a definitive role in the coordination and administration of existing community and hospital resources to optimize outcomes for all concerned.

• Critical Pathways: A Formula
   for Case Management Practice

The preoperative plan must consider a very tightly sequenced series of interdependent events — from initial scheduling, patient education, and testing to the patient's return to the home environment. Critical pathways for specific ambulatory surgical procedures assist in the patient care planning process

Figure 22-1. Ambulatory Surgery Program Advantages and Disadvantages

Hospital-based unit utilizing inpatient operating rooms (ORs) and a postanesthesia care unit

Advantages

1. Inpatient support services are always available.
2. Equipment, supplies, and staff are not duplicated.
3. Physicians work in the same ORs.
4. Operating room volumes utilize available space.
5. End-of-day "add-ons" can be performed.
6. Resources are immediately available for intraop emergency/complications.

Disadvantages

1. Communication and continuity of care are fragmented.
2. Paper flow is separated and occasionally misplaced.
3. It is expensive.
4. In an emergency inpatients take priority.
5. Patients often have difficulty finding the unit.

Hospital-based independent ORs and postanesthesia care

Advantages

1. Communication and continuity of care are improved.
2. Ancillary support services are available.
3. Outpatients are the priority.
4. Vacant rooms accommodate inpatient overflow.

Disadvantages

1. There's occasional duplication of staff, medical supplies, and equipment.
2. Scheduling conflicts occur due to shared equipment.
3. Physicians must travel between units when doing outpatient and inpatient surgery.
4. Conflicts with physician availability occur if physicians are scheduled in both locations.

(For both units, overnight stay is an option when the situation warrants.)

Freestanding unit

Advantages

1. The cost of the procedure is lower.
2. It offers a nonhospital environment and greater convenience.
3. There is greater focus on customer service.
4. It is more accessible for patients.

Disadvantages

1. Ancillary support services are limited.
2. Reimbursement is less; patients may have to pay out-of-pocket expenses.
3. Overnight stays are not an option, unless contracted.
4. The hours of operation are limited.
5. Patients with intraoperative complications may require transfer to a tertiary care facility.

and are a major component of program planning and successful outcomes. These critical pathways, often called *care mapping,* form the foundation of case management for the outpatient surgical patient.

Historically, critical pathways have been inpatient-oriented, problem-focused, driven by financial constraint, and designed to include care after discharge. In the outpatient setting (especially ambulatory surgery) the approach focuses instead on specific procedures and safe, timely patient processing and discharge. This strategy offers advantages in the ambulatory setting, because most encounters are for a single procedure or episode of illness. Procedure-specific pathways for outpatient surgery apply predefined surgical standards of care after individual patient needs are determined by the initial intake interview or referral. The encounter process is organized into five logical phases:

1. Preadmission
2. Admission/procedure
3. Postprocedure/observation
4. Discharge
5. Follow-up

Because the intensity of individual patients' needs are likely to vary at any one of these levels, so will resource utilization. Variables are likely to include patient age, overall health status, availability of family support systems, caregiver resources, and ultimate aftercare or home care requirements. Procedure- and encounter-specific critical pathways accommodate these variables and provide guidelines and controls for setting resource allocation priorities. When appropriately designed, individual pathways offer a documentation tool, a variance measurement, and an outcomes monitor.

In deploying a case management model, organizations should encourage an interdisciplinary approach to the development of critical pathways. The multidisciplinary entities should include admissions personnel, surgeons, perioperative clinical nursing staff, ancillary services personnel, anesthesiologists, social services personnel, and home care representatives. Because a primary role of critical pathways is to reduce variations in practice patterns, to optimize outcomes, and to improve communications to provide coordinated care, the integration of these disciplines is crucial. Thus, case management models can be set up for all types of ambulatory surgery programs emphasizing the importance of a high-quality care continuum in providing a competitive edge. Strategies for success include:

- Formation of a multidisciplinary team with a modular approach
- Well-defined scope of care
- Focused patient outcomes
- Achievement of service excellence

- Financial planning
- Evaluation of the patient's home environment
- Home health care arranged prior to surgery
- Networking of information systems
- Control of diagnostic testing and costs

Several considerations must be taken into account with regard to implementation. These include:

- Operational costs
- Staff (location, cross-training, rightsizing)
- Interaction with home health care or other community agencies
- Impact on how the patient is managed medically
- Transition from traditional care to case management

The case manager, familiar with the patient and aware of ongoing treatments and procedures, can eliminate duplicative or unnecessary diagnostic studies required for the current intervention. Cognizant of the patient's home environment and available support systems, the case manager can make necessary arrangements for staff, equipment, or medical supplies that may be needed postoperatively, well before the day of surgery. Health care assistance could be scheduled to begin immediately following the patient's discharge home.

• Successful Implementation

A question central to successful program implementation is: Who should be the case manager? The most logical choice is the ambulatory surgical nurse. A primary nursing model in a collaborative practice offers the best structure for ambulatory surgical case management. A collaborative, interdisciplinary practice with surgeons, anesthesiologists, nursing staff, ancillary services personnel, social workers, and home health contacts constitutes a complete, effective case management group. This group establishes specific criteria — or critical pathways — regarding the scope of care for certain targeted patient groups. The group negotiates and develops protocols for a formalized communication process and identifies the surgical nurse/case manager who will be responsible for the overall coordination of care. As case managers, ambulatory surgical nurses also can better fulfill one of the major roles of outpatient surgical care — patient education. Through their training and experience, surgical nurses are uniquely qualified to educate patients regarding their course of treatment. The consistent assignment of surgeons, nurses, and other case management group members throughout a single encounter allows a smooth transition for patient and family through all phases of planning, discharge, and continuing care.

When the need for surgical intervention is identified, the patient is scheduled for surgery and patient education is initiated. Patient education normally begins in the surgeon's office, with generic instruction regarding the scheduled procedure. Frequently, informational booklets are shared with the patient regarding surgery, hospital routine, anesthesia, and postoperative care. The surgeon notifies the case manager, who then begins the process of collecting pertinent information through an intake interview and a variety of communication systems, such as information systems, telephone calls to office staff and/or the patient and family, and previous medical records. This assessment mechanism familiarizes case managers with patients who have made repeat visits and allows them to obtain pertinent information regarding diagnostic studies that may have been done recently, thus preventing the patient from making additional trips to the hospital and accumulating unnecessary charges. Communication with the patient affords the patient the opportunity to ask specific questions about the perioperative process described in the booklet. The nurse then continues preop teaching and assessment regarding routine support systems or the need for home health care. Long-range programmatic design could add computer-generated mailings to ensure that each patient receives specific written instruction and education.[2]

The patient's financial status, insurance plan, preauthorization requirements, and additional coverage components should be evaluated early in the process so that appropriate intervention, second opinions, and negotiations for alternative arrangements can be accomplished well in advance of the scheduled procedure. Aftercare or discharge planning for the postoperative phase is begun well in advance of scheduled admission. Information obtained from the initial intake interview is expected to familiarize the case manager with the patient's home environment, prospective caregiver, and social structure in order to match these needs with anticipated procedural intervention and postoperative care requirements. Interaction with social services personnel is often necessary to arrange for additional support from nonhospital resources. Following surgery, once the patient is home, the case manager telephones the patient and/or the family to ensure that they understand and are complying with recommended treatment plans. The physician also is requested to evaluate continuing care requirements.

• Financial Incentives for Case Management

It has been forecasted that more than half of all hospital revenues will come from outpatient services by the year 2000. According to the managing director of Hamilton/KSA, surgical revenue has risen more significantly than any other component of outpatient revenues. Data compiled by Hamilton/KSA show that most hospitals are projecting between 70 and 80 percent growth in managed care revenue within the next three years.[3]

For reimbursement purposes, there are three types of ambulatory surgery programs. The first two are affiliated with hospitals: programs set within the hospital, and programs that are physically separate but part of the hospital organization. Freestanding ambulatory surgery centers are the third type. The facility type determines reimbursement by Medicare and other third-party payers. For hospital-related ambulatory surgery units, reimbursement is on a reasonable cost basis. This calculation includes the provider's direct and indirect costs that are necessary and appropriate for the efficient delivery of needed health care services to Medicare beneficiaries. For freestanding ambulatory surgical centers, Medicare reimburses facility fees and fees for professional services.

Professional fees are reimbursed in a similar manner to the methods employed above for payment of physician fees. The notable difference is the treatment of the facility fee. Medicare pays certified freestanding facilities a flat, prospectively determined rate for each covered procedure. No deductibles or copayments are imposed on beneficiaries for this type of service. Thus, outpatient surgical facilities embody the potential to achieve two of the government's primary goals: provision of high-quality services and reduction in health care costs.[4]

Medicare-certified facilities must meet the "conditions of coverage," which include standards relating to facilities' governing bodies and management, provision of surgical services, quality improvement programs, physical environments, medical staffs, nursing services, medical records, pharmaceutical services, and laboratory and radiologic services. Payment is made at prospectively determined rates per procedure as indicated on Medicare's approved List of Covered Procedures.[5] In November 1992, 900 additional procedures were approved and appended to this list. In light of these trends, hospital-related programs might wisely consider establishing ambulatory surgery as an alternative delivery system to maximize profits by decreasing inpatient utilization.

• Impact on Medical Management

The 1986 Omnibus Budget Reconciliation Act (OBRA) mandated creation of a prospective pricing system for selected ambulatory surgical procedures by October 1, 1987, generating Medicare's List of Covered Procedures. The recent expansion of the list is incentive for physicians to shift from the inpatient to the outpatient setting. When a physician accepts an outpatient surgical assignment, Medicare will pay 100 percent of reasonable charges instead of the usual 80 percent.[6]

When moving surgical inpatients to outpatient settings, some physicians still order a barrage of laboratory tests. Given the current legal environment, this practice reflects defensive medicine and often seeks to cover all (even remote) possible diagnostic abnormalities. These concerns are justifiable. When a suspected abnormality is not followed up, the physician's liability is at stake for misdiagnosis.[7] The critical pathway model allows case management groups to establish which perioperative tests are needed based on specific, predefined criteria. Further, when diagnostic test results are abnormal, a variance is documented and intervention is instituted as indicated. Thus, these mechanisms provide a protocol system that should allay physicians' fears of liability, effect cost control, and decrease practice variances.

Surgeons are very aware of the need to provide services in an outpatient setting whenever feasible, and for the most part they are eager to participate. Embracing today's attractive alternatives to the standard practitioner's fee-for-service, more and more physicians are joining independent practice associations (IPAs), health maintenance organizations (HMOs), and PHOs. This infrastructure will ultimately result in surgical case management. Collaboration among all caregivers will be essential for the smooth processing of patients throughout the perioperative experience. These alternative practices will require the surgeon to actively participate in case management, both professionally and financially.[8]

• Trends

Advances in anesthesia and in less-invasive surgical technology will continue to broaden the scope of ambulatory surgery in the future. Laser surgery, fiber optics, and high-tech catheters, in addition to systems providing continuous medication and outpatient monitoring, will reduce the need to hospitalize patients. Innovative concepts such as observative care and short-stay recovery care centers will further expand the purview of ambulatory surgery to include the American Society of Anesthesiologists' class I and II patients, who require nursing care and/or pain control overnight or up to 72 hours in a professional care environment. Figure 22-2 profiles the short stay or recovery care center concept that is emerging to serve patients who require professional care 23 to 72 hours after surgery.

The most prominent trend for ambulatory care in the 1990s will undoubtedly be that of providing care for subacute patients — those who are neither outpatient nor inpatient by virtue of the intensity of their services. The subacute, who usually require 24- to 72-hour stays, represent an enormous population of hospitalized inpatients. These patients will no doubt continue to grow in number as their payers are able to successfully contract with managed care providers for services at rates lower than those currently offered by hospitals.[9] By the early part of the next century, only the sickest patients will require inpatient hospitalization for surgery.[10]

Figure 22-2. Ambulatory Surgery Case Management Expanded to Recovery Care

---

Types of Recovery Care Centers

- Freestanding recovery care centers that contract with ambulatory surgery centers, hospital-affiliated and freestanding.
- Recovery care facility that is part of the ambulatory surgery center.
- Patient units within the hospital that are closed or have decreased inpatient stays are converted to 23- to 72-hour recovery care units.
- Medical hotel is a hotel environment for patients and families/friends. This type of facility could be a joint venture between two or more hospitals and/or surgicenters.

Advantages

- Most surgical inpatients qualify.
- Ancillary services are not needed.
- Revenue is available for hospitals with decreased patient census.
- Physicians and patients like them.

Disadvantages

- Arrangements for emergency care must be set up.
- State licensure and Medicare reimbursement are unavailable if the center is freestanding.
- Length of stay is restricted to 72 hours.

• Conclusion

The application of case management principles in ambulatory surgical care offers quality and cost containment benefits to patients, providers, and payers alike. Focused case management programs offer an opportunity for coordinated care and resource allocation that effectively support patients and families thrown into a complex environment for a stressful event. Similar to home health care models, case management in ambulatory surgery offers new opportunities for providing a continuum of care and serving a growing patient population that would not have been considered good ambulatory surgery candidates in the past. In short, ambulatory surgery case management embodies the total quality improvement concept, which spells the difference between merely meeting patients' needs and providing true quality care and patient satisfaction.

References

1. Berryman, J. M. Development and organization of outpatient surgery units: the hospital's perspective. *Urologic Clinics of North America* 14(1):1–9, Feb. 1987.

2. Miner, D. Preoperative outpatient education in the 1990's. *Nursing Management* 21(12):40–44, Dec. 1992.

3. Sabatino, F. What the upper Midwest knows: region leads the nation in net patient revenues. *Hospitals* 67(1):34–37, Jan. 1993.

4. Leap, J. M. The prospective payment system: its impact on ambulatory surgery programs. In: B. Breedlove, editor. *Successful Management of Ambulatory Surgery Programs.* Vol. 2. Atlanta, GA: American Health Consultants, 1985, pp. 103–7.

5. Romansky, M. A., and Millman, D. S. Regulatory and legal aspects of outpatient surgery. *Urologic Clinics of North America* 14(1):15–20, Feb. 1987.

6. Droste, T. Freestandings bound to gain under new PPS plan. *Hospitals* 61(13):60–61, July 1987.

7. Patterson, P. ASCs accepting older, higher risk patients. *OR Manager* 7(7):14–15, July 1991.

8. Burns, L. A. Business planning for ambulatory surgical services. *Surgical Clinics of North America* 67(4):709–19, Aug. 1987.

9. Matson, T. Ambulatory care to drive hospital services in 1990s. *Health Care Strategic Management* 9(3):16–18, Mar. 1991.

10. Riffer, J. Hernia surgery makes its move to outpatient settings. *Hospitals* 60(8):79, Apr. 1986.

Chapter 23

Case Management Model: Primary Care

Carol Wilson Garvey, MD

• Introduction

Any implementation of health reform will necessarily include various models of primary care case management that typify the virtues and practice ideals of primary and preventive medicine. This agenda is ensured by the acknowledged need for the consistent medical oversight and management of patient care in a manner that promotes quality and reduces cost. As the ultimate manager of medical care, the attending primary care physician plays an obvious and key role in achieving this goal.

Managed care initiatives are the most familiar of these prototypes. Recently, some progressive state entitlement programs began to enlist the primary care management strategy in the assignment of primary care physicians to underserved patient populations. This approach is a response to the need for improved access to the health care continuum, reduced utilization of high-cost emergency departments (EDs) for episodic and chronic care, and consistent, coordinated medical care and resource allocation. Unfortunately, a number of barriers inhibit the logical execution of this process. In a nation where more than two-thirds of practicing physicians are specialists or subspecialists, there is a painfully obvious undersupply of primary care practitioners to meet the growing need for comprehensive case management and coordination.

Compounding the physician supply problem is the difficulty of gaining access to the most appropriate level of care and caregiver in today's jumble of alternatives. This nation's health care system continues to feed more and more subacute patients into the ambulatory care arena yet provides little guidance for the patient without a physician or, worse, without insurance. Even the local ED is relatively inaccessible at some facilities where overcrowding and advanced triage systems disallow treatment for nonemergency conditions. Further, the episodic care received in the ED breaks the continuity of care for many patients who seek it for chronic illness. Without proper follow-up care by a physician, the patient may have to return to the ED again and again. Further, if the ED is in a separate facility without access to previous medical records, diagnosis and treatment may be misdirected or duplicated at considerable cost to the payer.

The primary care case management model addresses the issues of cost, quality, and access by entrusting patients to the expert guidance of their primary care providers — physicians in general or family practice, internal medicine, pediatrics, and, in some instances, obstetrics/gynecology. This chapter describes the benefits of the primary care model and the barriers to its implementation. It also addresses the model's financial incentives and its impact on medical management.

• Benefits of Primary Care Case Management

Primary care case management emphasizes the physician's role as the best-qualified medical case manager. High-quality, continuous health care co-ordinated by a single provider reduces unnecessary hospitalization and inappropriate use of system resources. Additionally, it supports the goals of health care reform by reducing service fragmentation, slowing cost escalation, and addressing the fundamental service needs of the majority of patients.

The primary care physician's office gives patients a "medical home" where basic health care services are provided and copies of all medical records are stored. Normally, health screening (routine checkups), preventive services (such as immunizations), and most sick care are provided in the outpatient setting. Because the primary care physician often is responsible for several family members, he or she is able to understand a patient's illness in the context of its repercussions not only for the patient but also for the patient's family. The physician is also more likely to be aware of the family's socioeconomic situation, and thus can adjust treatments and resources to match the family's ability to cope with the illness financially.

Most primary care practices provide 24-hour-a-day telephone access for optimal patient management. All visits to specialists or EDs should occur only if the primary care physician has determined that this is the most appropriate approach to treatment. Conditions or circumstances that merit treatment outside the primary care setting may be determined either by direct physical examination or via a telephone evaluation. Properly used, the primary care case management model eliminates the provision of unnecessary services and is responsive to the psychosocial as well as the physical needs of the patient.

As an example, a primary care physician's examination of a 10-month-old child with a fever of 104 degrees shows the child to be apathetic and floppy. The mother gives a sketchy history and says little in general. A physician who knows the family from prior encounters may recognize that this child is apathetic and relatively floppy even when well and that this mother, although not verbal, is capable of caring for an ill child and has done so successfully with other children in the family. In the absence of specific alarming physical or laboratory findings, the primary care physician may send the child home with instructions for follow-up care. However, an ED physician, to whom the mother and child are unknown, may feel compelled to perform a battery of tests, perform a lumbar puncture, and even hospitalize the child because of the possibility of meningitis, having no way to gauge current findings against the child's normal status.

This example illustrates how the primary case management model has potential for addressing other issues currently plaguing the health care system. The issues in this case would include misutilization of the ED; duplication and overuse of services, diagnostics, and prescriptions; and higher rates of inpatient hospitalization.

A number of state entitlement programs are following the path of the primary care case management model, linking Medicaid recipients with physician providers. Kentucky, Utah, Michigan, and Colorado have implemented primary care programs. Maryland and others have recently followed suit by activating Access to Care programs of similar design. Independent surveys from participating states indicate generally positive responses from patients, payers, and physician providers alike. Physicians find that such programs ensure quality of care, strengthen doctor–patient relationships, and more effectively utilize scarce health care resources. These programs are intended to decrease inappropriate utilization of the health care system and to ensure access to preventive and continuing primary health care. Although the individual state models vary in their perspectives and components, they share a common goal: to achieve cost-effective care management. However, although these pilots have set the stage for development of such endeavors in the ambulatory care arena, there are certain formidable barriers to implementing such programs.

• Barriers to Implementation

Key to the success of primary care case management is the availability of providers in general or family practice, internal medicine, pediatrics, and obstetrics/gynecology. Unfortunately, the dearth of such providers and declines in the number of physicians entering primary care practice may severely limit applicability of this model of care despite its universal appeal. Such a model works as well in an urban or rural community health center as it does in a private suburban practice, conferring both quality and cost-control benefits to medical care management in any practice setting.

Physician education will make or break the future of primary care case management. Medical schools certainly influence their students' choices to pursue primary care or specialty practice, and the government already is intervening to ensure that schools quickly and successfully encourage more students to choose primary care. In the near future, governmental disincentives such as limits on financial support for specialty training programs are likely.

The perceived competitive threat from alternate providers or "physician extenders" such as nurse practitioners, nurse midwives, and physician assistants has limited the potential for collaboration in private settings. In some publicly supported community and migrant health centers, academic facilities, and closed-panel health maintenance organizations (HMOs), the primary care provider is a physician extender or nurse practitioner who functions independently but in consultative collaboration with the physician. A personal disadvantage for the primary care-oriented physician in this type of practice arrangement is the absence of close personal relationships with patients—one of the rewards of being a family physician. Most states, including New York, New Jersey, Ohio, and California, bar nurses from practicing independently. On the other hand, in Arizona, Alaska, and five other states, nurses own and manage medical clinics. For example, Carondelet Nursing Network in Tucson, Arizona, operates 17 primary care clinics and provides home care for the chronically ill. Medicare is piloting a program that allows nurses to act as the primary care gatekeeper for patients without a primary care physician. Both collaborative and independent nursing-based primary care case management models have achieved cost-effective care delivery and high levels of patient satisfaction, while providing care for greater numbers of patients.

• Financial Incentives

If effective primary care case management demands an educational pipeline that produces an adequate flow of physicians and alternative providers, it also demands purchasers who will accept a diversity of medical providers, settings, and financing mechanisms. Purchasers also must be convinced that the primary care medical home model has been adjusted to serve their regional geography, demography, and resource availability.

For payers, the financial incentives of a primary care model of health care delivery are many. Preventive and health screening initiatives are of considerable value in documented long-term savings through the early diagnosis and treatment of illness. A second and major benefit of focused primary care management is reduced utilization of high-cost emergency services and unnecessary specialist visits. The enrollment of patients who consistently use their selected or assigned primary care providers to direct and manage their care offers significant economic advantages for private industry, shared federal- and state-funded (Medicaid) programs, and federal (Medicare) programs alike.

Financial incentives for physicians are more complex. Some physicians make a conscious decision to avoid entering primary care practice in favor of more remunerative subspecialties that will allow them to more quickly pay off heavy financial debts incurred in medical school and practice start-up. For those who choose primary care, the financial aspects of its practice affect physicians and their patients in various ways; for example, a patient's insurance or lack of insurance may affect the thoroughness and thus the expense of a primary care encounter.

For example, for many physicians, optimal medical management of a urinary tract infection includes urinalysis, culture, and antibiotic sensitivity testing prior to treatment and again after the treatment course is completed. An uninsured patient without obvious complications might be adequately, though not ideally, managed with examination, initial urinalysis (presumably confirmed as suspected infection by the presence of bacteria, leukocytes, and often red blood cells), empiric antibiotic treatment, and no follow-up lab work unless symptoms persist.

Although fee-for-service physicians have felt political heat for the potential abuses of overutilization and self-referral, both the public and its elected officials appear oblivious to the strong incentives for abuse inherent in capitated payment schemes in arrangements such as independent practice associations (IPAs). Inferior plan structuring that results in insufficient capitation payments or rates may preclude the provision of preventive care to patients, and financial penalties for "excessive" referrals eventually may lead to more hospitalizations for more acute illnesses. The insurer who fails to provide cost-effective preventive services passes along a greater financial burden that someone else down the line must hoist.

For example, a low capitation rate, annually amounting to less than the cost of a normal physical exam, may discourage a patient's IPA provider from ever doing a Pap smear. Should the patient change insurers with a geographic move or a new job (as is likely within a decade), the cost of treating a subsequent cervical carcinoma will be borne by the new insurer, not by the IPA that initially failed to detect it.

A number of factors may undermine the ability of primary care case management to limit medical expenditures. These include:

- The physician's drive to fully understand the causes and monitor the effects of a patient's illness through frequent lab, X-ray, and other testing
- The patient's anxiety and desire to have specific data and complete explanations
- The patient's sense of entitlement to the latest technology (for example, magnetic resonance imaging for diagnosis of headaches)
- The physician's fear of malpractice suits if "everything" is not done

There are additional factors that interfere with the effectiveness and appropriateness of primary care case management under nonrestrictive insurance plans. These include:

- The use of EDs or walk-in clinics for routine or nonurgent care outside normal medical office hours
- Self-referral to specialists without consulting the primary care physicians (for example, a referral to a rheumatologist or orthopedist for arthritis, which often can be handled by a primary care physician)
- Doctor shopping for controlled drugs or to obtain care for conditions not disclosed to the family's primary care provider (for example, symptoms thought to be related to an illicitly acquired sexually transmitted disease)

• Impact on Medical Management and Confounding Factors

A clearly identified primary health care provider orchestrates all care by other practitioners. Conflicting recommendations by consulting specialists are resolved by the primary provider, based on information gained through direct communication or examination of the patient.

Although primary medical management ideally addresses the entire continuum of medical care, encompassing office visits and procedures, house calls, acute hospital care, and home and aftercare, evolving reimbursement policies threaten the integrity of the comprehensive model. Recent Medicare policy precludes payments to both an internist and an internal medicine subspecialist for hospital visits to the same patient on the same day. Thus, a primary care internist who feels that cardiology consultation is required for optimal care of a medically unstable patient may not be reimbursed for visiting the patient on the day of the cardiologist's visit. As in Great Britain's National Health Service, current Health Care Financing Administration (HCFA) policy encourages office-based generalists to terminate their medical care of hospitalized patients and transfer them to hospital-based specialists. Although this policy may have been intended as a federal cost-saving measure, it may be detrimental to the patient's psychological and/or clinical well-being.

Intricate insurance mechanisms often demand that a primary physician articulate a patient treatment plan for presentation and scrutiny prior to payment approval by a designated reimbursement agency. This engenders frustration for the physician who, though forced to spend more and more time on administrative chores, is chastised for having such a high billing rate. The treatment plan format familiar to nursing and social service personnel has not traditionally been taught to medical students, and the time sacrificed for its completion appears to many physicians to impede rather than facilitate patient care. This bureaucratic burden appears to be an inevitable requirement and consequence of the managed care concept. A newer generation of physicians may find it more palatable, if not more productive.

Escalating government demands for accountability in areas such as laboratory management (application of the Federal Clinical Laboratories Improvement Act [CLIA-88] to all physicians' offices in 1992) and personnel safety (1992 Occupational Safety and Health Administration [OSHA] regulations for protection of medical personnel from hepatitis B and AIDS) have driven many physicians to consider restructuring their practices. As administrative expenses climb, the smaller office practice loses its financial viability. In the coming decades, the majority of physicians are likely to be employees of larger organizations rather than individual practitioners or entrepreneurs. It is unfortunate but true that, under these circumstances, the closeness of many primary care physician–patient relationships will likely diminish, because the hand that feeds the physician will be the employer's rather than the patient's.

Tales of patients becoming "lost in the system" are heard with increasing frequency as more complex systems of care evolve. The role of the primary medical care practitioner is at once more crucial and more difficult to achieve than in previous decades. A substantial increase in numbers of primary care physicians will be required if patients are to retain access to a knowledgeable advocate as they navigate the medical maze of diagnostic and therapeutic options.

• Practice Parameters, Costs, and the Primary Care Physician

The impending era of practice parameters presents new opportunities and dilemmas. Formulaic or "cookbook" responses to the intricacies of psychic and somatic dysfunctions are being vigorously resisted by many physicians. However, the inevitable implementation of this approach, based on outcomes research, may allow for substantial reductions in physician liability judgments and thus pave the way for major tort reform.

Current liability costs burden not only practicing physicians but also physician training programs. Although the effect on medical school costs is less direct, overall physician education costs may be significantly reduced if the use of practice parameters and guidelines lower schools' liability and practice costs.

Practice parameters are promoted as potential instruments for limiting "unnecessary" testing and procedures, but as with the quality assurance measures that preceded them by several decades, they actually may increase practice costs. First, practice guidelines may recommend interventions that are not currently universally ordered by physicians, and, second, monitoring for compliance will be a necessary and costly component of implementation.

However, there also is a positive outcome of practice parameters. They may empower primary care providers to embark on the initial evaluation of problems for which they previously might have sought early specialist intervention. Should management under the parameters prove straightforward, the need for costly consultation may be averted. Such an outcome may strengthen the role of the primary care physician and enhance his or her satisfaction in assuming primary responsibility for patients.

• Monitoring of Office-Based Primary Care Quality

Although internal and external approaches to the direct monitoring of office-based practice are still in the embryonic stage, indirect measures are plentiful. Indirect quality monitors include:

- Credentialing by hospitals for admission privileges
- Quality assurance reviews of patient admissions to hospitals
- Credentialing by specialty societies, including periodic reexamination every seven years by the American College of Family Practice (ACFP)
- Credentialing by state licensing bodies, often including continuing medical education requirements

Direct measures include the self-administered office chart reviews required by the American Board of Family Practice (ABFP) prior to each recredentialing exam and Medicare's recent computerized analyses of office visit levels of care. In an innovative HMO such as Harvard Community Health Plan, extensive quality review activities are possible through computerized evaluation of documented follow-up (or lack of follow-up) for laboratory abnormalities. However, this highly valuable approach depends on a fully computerized medical record, which is rarely found in office practice and, when found, is not always well utilized for quality monitoring.

Although adherence to Lawrence Weed's problem-oriented medical record (POMR) format[1] facilitates review of office records, the illegibility of many records precludes effective evaluation. It is unlikely that direct monitoring will be feasible until and unless the full computerization of records becomes inexpensive and universal. The question also must be asked whether, in view of the large number of indirect quality measures available, routine direct monitoring of office care quality will be either cost-effective or appropriate.

• Expanding Primary Care Resources

As the nation wrestles with medical care cost containment, the need for more primary care case managers is apparent. Medical schools enlarged their classes at the urging of the federal government in the 1970s, and the number of physicians has further grown with the steady influx of foreign medical graduates.

However, as mentioned earlier, the number of physicians entering primary care has remained small. Although educational support through programs such as the National Health Service Corps provides incentive to medical students to enter primary care, additional measures appear to be necessary. Reducing the cost of medical education would defray the debt burdens, which often are responsible for driving students into the higher-paying specialties.

The key players in redirecting educational resources toward primary care are the American Association of Medical Colleges (AAMC) and the American Medical Association (AMA). Should these associations fail in their efforts to effect a significant and prompt increase in primary care physicians, the federal government can be expected to direct resources away from specialty programs and require medical schools to meet minimum primary care graduate quotas.

Adequate primary care reimbursement through Medicare, Medicaid, and other federal or state physician reimbursement plans must be ensured if medical students are to consider careers in primary care. The 1992 implementation of HCFA's resource-based relative value scale (RBRVS) for Medicare reimbursement reduced many specialists' fees by as much as 50 percent over a four-year time span but failed to deliver the promised significant increases to primary care physicians.

• Conclusion

The effectiveness of the primary care physician as medical care case manager is indisputable among educators, payers, and most patients. Over the next decade, as medicine becomes more technologically complex and health care delivery is restructured, primary care physicians will perform a major role in coordinating clinical services for the patients entrusted to their care. The role and practice of the primary physician will evolve in response to the managed care pressures of health financing reform. Whether in private practice or as an employee of a health maintenance organization, the primary care physician will function as gatekeeper to the system. Additional nursing-based or physician extender models will proliferate in regions without adequate physician supply.

Efforts to improve access to primary care for all patients, to reduce costs and eliminate duplicative services, and to achieve continuity of care in a fragmented health care system will keep the nation's health care leaders and federal and state legislators busy for years to come. The real challenge lies in determining the best mechanisms and practices to cultivate a sufficient and equitably distributed supply of the health care system's most valuable provider — the primary care physician. Without a strong core of primary care physicians, any attempted health care reforms will be in grave jeopardy from the very start.

Note

1. Weed, L. L. Medical records that guide and teach. *New England Journal of Medicine* 278(11):593–600, 1968; and 278(12):652–57, 1968. The problem-oriented medical record (POMR) approach developed in the 1960s by Dr. Weed and taught by nearly all U.S. medical schools since then requires that physicians and other health care providers write orderly and focused notes on each of a patient's medical problems according to the following outline:

   - Subjective: The problem as described by the patient or history giver
   - Objective: The objective findings on the physical exam and any administered tests
   - Assessment: The provider's diagnosis (definite or provisional) at the time the note is written
   - Plan: The provider's intended actions based on the assessment and possibly including further diagnostic testing, medication, patient education, referral, and/or return visits

Part III

A Selective Annotated Bibliography of the Case Management Literature

David P. Moxley, PhD

• Introduction to the Bibliography

The literature of case management reflects the growing diversity and complexity of human service and health care practice. Beginning as a relatively sparse selection of literature in the late 1970s and early 1980s, case management literature has expanded as this form of practice has continued to become rooted in human service and health care delivery systems. Like any literature on new forms of practice, case management literature initially addressed the need for case management and prescribed its impact on various social problems.

In the wake of deinstitutionalization, however, case management was identified as a front line service in organizing and integrating services for the most vulnerable of our citizens including people experiencing developmental disabilities, serious mental illness, or problems associated with aging and chronic illness. Thus, it is not surprising to find a great deal of the literature on case management focusing on mental health, disability, or aging issues. Case management also was linked to the growing quality of service movement in the United States, and so we see in the literature, beginning in the mid-1980s, the use of case management as a means for promoting the quality of health and human services. A third perspective on the use of case management also is reflected in the literature on the cost containment movement. Much of this literature is grounded in case management as utilization and risk management within the framework of managed care.

The purpose of this bibliography is to offer readers a listing and an overview of selected literature in the broad field of case management. Of course, the bibliography is not exhaustive. It does offer readers a foundation that can serve them well in building their own broad and/or specific understanding of this field. The organizational scheme of the bibliography is quite simple. The first section reviews books in the field that identify the multiple and diverse applications of case management models, technology, and program development factors. The second section reviews journal literature that identifies several of the major issues facing case management.

• Book-Length Treatments of Case Management

General Treatment and Survey of Case Management

Moxley, D. P. *The Practice of Case Management.* Newbury Park, CA: Sage Publications, 1989 (155 pages).

> This book offers a general perspective on case management practice. Moxley develops a transdisciplinary model of case management that identifies its various functions and activities including assessment of needs, services, and supports; the development of care plans; case management intervention; and monitoring and evaluation. Moxley conceives the focus of case management to be the creation of a "client support network" involving the integration and coordination of self care, professional care, and mutual care. The book offers an introduction to case management practice but fails to offer a critical perspective on this form of practice.

Raiff, N., and Shore, B. *Advanced Case Management: New Strategies for the Nineties.* Newbury Park, CA: Sage Publications, 1993 (190 pages).

> This book captures the state of the art in case management practice and offers the reader an understanding of the plethora of practices and innovations that have emerged in the late 1980s and early 1990s. The authors conceive of case management as a constellation of various program forms ranging from rather simple arrangements to very complex ones. Advanced case management is seen as a means of mustering an array of services to address the needs of the most vulnerable clients — those individuals who present complex needs and situations and who, as a result, require well integrated and coordinated service and support responses. This book has many strengths including its identification of critical service and design variables. The authors offer an intriguing "metamodel" of case management that integrates traditional functions with cutting edge issues like cultural competence, consumer empowerment, clinical case management, and multidisciplinary practice. The authors, however, do not examine the actual merit and worth of case management.

Rothman, J. *Guidelines for Case Management: Putting Research to Professional Use.* Itasca, IL: Peacock Publishers, 1993 (127 pages).

The author has undertaken a very important service for those professionals who are interested in case management from a practice perspective. Rothman has critically examined the knowledge base of the field and identifies generalizations from the literature and related action guidelines that can be used to design case management interventions, develop case management programs, and evaluate the impact and effectiveness of case management. Generalizations and action guidelines are organized according to case management practice roles, linking clients to informal supports, linking clients to formal agency supports, staffing and training, and evaluation of case management effectiveness. A final compendium summarizes specific action guidelines. For health care professionals looking to base case management program design and implementation on the knowledge base of the field this book is an excellent resource. However, Rothman does not really examine specific models of case management.

Weil, M., Karls, J., and associates. *Case Management in Human Service Practice.* San Francisco: Jossey-Bass, 1985 (407 pages).

This work is one of the earliest book-length treatments of case management and the authors offer an excellent overview and survey of case management that remains relevant to this day. The book is organized into three major sections with the first section addressing the knowledge base of the field, the second section examining the application of case management to specific populations, and the third section examining practice implications. The second section of the book is very valuable since it surveys the range of case management applications to the needs of various vulnerable populations or to specific social problems including child welfare, aging, health care, mental illness, developmental disabilities, and physical disabilities. The book is a well integrated and comprehensive treatment of case management theory, history, practice, and applications.

Case Management in Mental Health, Developmental Disabilities, and Rehabilitation

Harris, M., and Bachrach, L., editors. *Clinical Case Management.* San Francisco: Jossey-Bass, 1988 (101 pages).

This book addresses case management and serious mental illness. The perspective of the book is that serious mental illness requires the integration of clinical and service coordination and integration activities in order to be truly responsive to the needs of individuals who are coping with persistent disabling psychiatric conditions. The editors integrate clinical perspectives into the formation of case management relationships, case management service planning, family involvement, and the creation of linkages between case management and inpatient care, housing, and continuity of care. A chapter on financing case management in order to achieve desired service goals is an important contribution of this volume. The strength of this book lies in its portrayal of a distinctive model of case management in the field of serious mental illness. Yet, the authors place so much emphasis on clinical mental health care that the community support aspects of case management tend to be overlooked.

Levine, I., and Fleming, M. *Human Resource Development: Issues in Case Management.* Washington, DC: National Institute of Mental Health, no date (86 pages).

This monograph represents one of the earliest treatments of case management in the field of mental health. In the preface, the authors define case management in the context of accountability and they view it as "a method of fixing responsibility for systems coordination with one individual, who works with a given client in accessing necessary services." The strength of this volume lies in its presentation of various models of case management including the generalist approach, specialist approach, therapist–case manager model, family model, psychosocial rehabilitation model, and supportive care model. The authors anticipated the involvement of volunteers and family members in case management service delivery. The volume also is distinctive in its efforts to address issues pertaining to the configuration and development of the human resource dimension of case management.

Linz, M., McAnally, P., and Wieck, C. *Case Management: Historical, Current, and Future Perspectives.* Cambridge, MA: Brookline Books, 1989 (168 pages).

The issue-based character of this volume makes it an important contribution to the literature of case management in the field of developmental disabilities. The chapters, written by national leaders in the developmental disabilities movement, address issues that are often overlooked by functional orientations to case management. The authors explore community building, the politics of case management implementation, the integration of services, and the application of case management to different phases of the life cycle. Family and consumer perspectives are explored as are perspectives on aspects of social policy, law, and the implementation of case management within local service systems. A chapter on "A new way of thinking for case managers" addresses issues that are very relevant to changing the culture of health and human service delivery for people with developmental disabilities. These issues also are very relevant to organizing services and support for people coping with serious and life-threatening illness.

Roessler, R. T., and Rubin, S. E. *Case Management and Rehabilitation Counseling: Procedures and Techniques.* Baltimore: University Park Press, 1982 (205 pages).

The authors take a very traditional approach to case management within the context of the role of vocational rehabilitation counselors. Emphasis is placed on the role and functions of rehabilitation counselors and their use of case management to organize more effective services for their clients with challenges arising out of disability. Considerable attention is paid to the organization and coordination of assessments and evaluations including medical, psychological, and vocational ones. In addition, attention is paid to developing individualized rehabilitation programs. The authors do not address the more macro and service system dynamics of case management, nor do they address the interdisciplinary interface of vocational rehabilitation with community support, health care, housing, or educational systems.

Sanborn, C. J., editor. *Case Management in Mental Health Services.* New York City: Haworth, 1983 (198 pages).

Despite the author's emphasis on the application of case management to mental health services, this pioneering volume frames case management as a generic human service concept that is relevant when confronting issues of support and service coordination created by serious disability. The chapters composing this volume address the rationale for case management, systemic and organizational issues, legal and ethical issues, the preparation of case managers, and the application of case management to rehabilitation. Three case studies demonstrate the application of case management to mental health services, developmental disabilities, and welfare. The author anticipated many of the case management themes that were to become visible in the late 1980s (for example, consumer-driven case management). This book represents a core text of the field and offers readers a historical perspective on the introduction of case management to health and human service systems.

Surber, R. W., editor. *Clinical Case Management: A Guide to Comprehensive Treatment of Serious Mental Illness.* Newbury Park, CA: Sage, 1994 (275 pages).

This volume is a guide to the integration of clinical mental health perspectives with case management. The aim is to create a more relevant service for people with serious mental illness than what is typically available through case management forms that emphasize brokerage or service coordination. Sixteen chapters cover the range of issues created by serving people with serious mental illness through a clinical case management approach. A section on clinical case management themes includes chapters on clinical case management as an approach to care and the engagement of families and members of informal support systems. A second section addresses traditional functions of assessment, treatment planning, linkage, and advocacy. A third section covers a range of specific treatment issues including substance abuse, working with people who present personality disorders, intervening into problematic behaviors, and supporting client goal attainment. Absent from this volume are critical perspectives relating to case management as social control, the use of case management to address legal issues created by mental illness, the interface between case management and the criminal justice system, and the use of case management as an alternative to inpatient commitment. These omissions reduce the comprehensiveness of the volume.

Case Management in Aging, Long-Term Care, and Home Care Service Systems

Applebaum, R., and Austin, C. *Long Term Case Management: Design and Evaluation.* New York City: Springer, 1990 (179 pages).

This book will be of primary interest to health care providers engaged in the design and evaluation of quality case management programs and systems. The volume incorporates three major parts that organize nine chapters. The first four chapters focus on the design of case management. The chapter on basic concepts identifies three major case management models involving brokering, service management, and managed care. The chapter on case management design options addresses the interface between case management and the local service system, tasks and functions of case managers, staffing and professionalization issues, configuration of the program, authority of case managers, interface of the case management system with the health care sector, timing of case management intervention, caseload parameters, and the case manager–client relationship. The second part of the book offers perspectives on evaluative and monitoring approaches and specific strategies for implementing quality assurance. The third part of the book examines the planning of case management and examines issues created by context including program, agency, local delivery systems, and state and federal policies. The strength of this volume lies in its incorporation of empirical data, reviews of demonstration projects, and analysis of specific service programs.

Bogdonoff, M. D., Hughes, S. L., Weissert, W. G., and Paulsen, E. *The Living-at-Home Program: Innovations in Service Access and Case Management.* New York City: Springer, 1991 (318 pages).

The authors offer readers an in-depth review of a program designed specifically to assist individuals who are aging with cost-effective supports designed to enable them to remain in home settings. The first section devotes four chapters to describing and documenting the program as a model. Background issues on home care for elders who are frail, an overview of the program, a review of the national evaluation of the model, and the use of home-based care to achieve cost-effectiveness are reviewed. The second section of the book examines specific issues and the experiences of exemplar demonstrations in relationship to these issues which include interagency cooperation, housing innovations, innovations in neighborhood outreach, outreach to ethnic populations, expanding social services and supports, and financing of services. This volume is an excellent resource not only on this specific demonstration and evaluation of home-based care but also on the use of access strategies, service expansion, and case management.

Kane, R. A., and Caplan, A. L., editors. *Ethical Conflicts in the Management of Home Care: The Case Manager's Dilemma.* New York City: Springer, 1993 (276 pages).

The ethical dimensions of case management in home-based care are examined in this volume which offers an excellent resource to practitioners, administrators, and policy makers involved in case management service delivery. The book grew out of the experiences and technical assistance work of the University of Minnesota National Long Term Care Decisions Resource Center with state and community programs serving the elderly. The practical and valid character of the volume is found in its content, issues, case studies, and examples. Ethical conflicts inherent to case management are identified including risk management, value conflicts between family members and elderly clients, protection of privacy, the allocation of scarce resources, the relationship between client preferences and costs, and the fair treatment of vendors. Much of the content of the core chapters address these conflicts or ones that are directly related to issues of fairness, equality, equity, and social control.

Quinn, J. *Successful Case Management in Long Term Care.* New York City: Springer, 1993 (157 pages).

This volume examines case management in the context of long-term care. The author offers an overview of the long-term care service system and addresses aging in the United States, long-term care policy, and experiences from demonstration projects. The author then offers specific practices and guidelines for assessment, care planning, and monitoring and evaluation. Specific issues pertaining to planning are given attention including ethical issues, conservatorship, nursing home placement, health problems, and informal supports. The final chapter is devoted to specific practice models. The author reviews a freestanding case management agency, special units, multifunction agencies, the consortium model, and an insurance case management model. The strength of this volume lies in the author's identification of these various models. However, the brief and limited attention she gives to each model reduces the richness that this volume can offer to health care practitioners seeking specific information and data on how to develop, implement, and evaluate these various approaches to case management.

Quinn, J., Segal, J., Raisz, H., and Johnson, C., editors. *Coordinating Community Services for the Elderly.* New York City: Springer, 1982 (125 pages).

This book represents a documentary overview and analysis of one of the first applications of case management and service coordination to the enhancement and cost containment of service delivery to persons who experience health and mental health problems as a result of aging. The volume reports on experiences learned by the staff of the Triage project, which was funded as a Medicare demonstration project in the late 1970s. The purpose of the project was to offer and test a client-centered approach to community service delivery to compensate for functional dependencies as a result of aging. The early chapters of the book capture the rationale of the project and the design and implementation of a client-centered system of service delivery. Other chapters focus on the financing and delivery aspects of the project including the use of waivers, holistic assessment, and service coordination and monitoring. The book is very relevant to health care practitioners who want to understand the historical context of current state-of-the-art delivery of long-term care, the diversion of older adults from unnecessary institutionalization, cost containment strategies in long-term care, and the integration of supports and services into an accessible framework of high-quality service provision.

Steinberg, R. M., and Carter, G. W. *Case Management and the Elderly: A Handbook for Planning and Administering Programs.* Lexington, MA: Lexington Books, 1983 (211 pages).

This is one of the early works anticipating the emergence of case management as a set of service delivery and organizational strategies in the 1980s. The data for the book were obtained through the authors' research on case management approaches, activities, and programs sponsored by the Older Americans Act. The book organizes these data in a qualitative, practical, and accessible manner so that models, programmatic procedures, state-of-the-art practices, and program development guidelines are clearly identified within a framework of choice. The authors organize the content so that it is amenable to program development. Emphasis is placed on alternative conceptions of the client service pathway, organizational factors and influences, enhancing the service system, maintaining coordination efforts, financing, human resource development, practice issues, and information management and evaluation. Readers who are interested in the design of case management policies and practices will want to review this book. Despite its relative age, the book remains vital to the improvement of our service systems for people who are aging and to the creation of more effective case management systems.

Case Management in the Context of Professional Discipline

Del Togno-Armanasco, V., Hopkin, L. A., and Harter, S. *Collaborative Nursing Case Management: A Handbook for Development and Implementation.* New York City: Springer, 1993 (183 pages).

This volume addresses the distinctive contribution made to case management by acute care nurses. The authors offer a patient care model of case management that responds to a changing policy context in which a "consumer focus" must be maintained despite an increasing emphasis placed on efficiency, regulatory change, and the emergence of new managed-care models. Case management is seen by the authors as the "coordination of the patient's care process" and they assert that it must be undertaken in collaboration with other professional providers and care providers. The content of the book is based on the authors' experience in developing and implementing a nursing case management service at a hospital based in Tucson, Arizona. Eight chapters address basic program development issues including plan development, the integration of the program into the continuum of care, the involvement of "key players," the development of staff, and the maintenance and evaluation of the program. A final chapter addresses the costs and benefits of this model program. The appendices offer specific applications of the model to several different acute health problems.

Rose, S. M. *Case Management and Social Work Practice.* New York City: Longman, 1992 (309 pages).

This volume focuses on case management as a core social work practice function. It offers a comprehensive overview of social work's view of case management and its implementation in mental health, health care, long-term care, and in emerging problem areas. The strength of this volume is its integration of many different perspectives on the application of case management undertaken by social workers. The book contains an overview of specific case management standards formulated by the National Association of Social Workers and the American Hospital Association. In the section on mental health, diverse case management approaches are identified and reviewed including clinical case management, community support, assertive community treatment, and the use of strengths perspectives. In the section on health care, issues raised by DRGs for the implementation of case management are identified. An encompassing theme is the diversity of case management within social work practice and the distinctive role of social work professionals in developing and delivering relevant case management services. This volume is very relevant to those readers who are interested in formulating case management responses with social work as the lead discipline. A weakness of this volume lies in the absence of interdisciplinary and transdisciplinary content which creates limitations for the use of this book in the design of case management efforts involving a broad range of disciplines.

Vourlekis, B. S., and Greene, R. R., editors. *Social Work Case Management.* New York City: Aldine de Gruyter, 1992 (199 pages).

This volume on case management and social work integrates the role of social work in the delivery of essential case management functions including outreach, assessment, care planning, service linkage, service implementation and monitoring, advocacy, and evaluation and quality assurance. The distinctive character of this volume lies in its linking case management functions to specific service delivery challenges, service populations, and specialized service contexts. The chapters are devoted to issues such as the case management assessment of infants with disabling conditions, care planning for children with HIV infection, the use of adult protective services case management with clients who are developmentally disabled, and family advocacy in the military. The authors communicate the diversity and flexibility of case management and the involvement of professionally prepared social workers in a multitude of efforts designed to create responsive human services for individuals, families, and groups. The first two chapters offer a framework for the distinctive contributions that social workers can make to case management efforts.

• Case Management Policy, Program, and Service Delivery Issues

The Issue of Advocacy and Resource Management

Dill, A. Issues in case management for the chronically mentally ill. In: D. Mechanic, editor. *Improving Mental Health Services: What the Social Sciences Can Tell Us.* San Francisco: Jossey-Bass, 1987.

> Dill asserts that there is an inherent conflict in the roles of many case managers due to the necessity of integrating into case management formal organizational activities with those of primary group affiliation. The case manager, according to Dill, represents to the client formal organizational and rationalized functions including assessor of needs, planner of services, counselor, and monitor of services. However, in many definitions of case management, the incumbent in this role must also passionately represent the needs of consumers within the service system and form a strong and perhaps personalized bond with the consumer. These different role activities may conflict in practice and create ethical dilemmas for the case manager and confusion for the consumer. The case manager may need to represent a neutral stance when interacting with the consumer such as when serving as a therapist but may need to argue and "sell" the consumer's needs or perspectives within the context of administrative hearings, intake situations, or advocacy situations. Dill raises an important issue of whether the role of case manager is a formal one or an informal one. Attempts to integrate the two may create a great deal of role conflict and strain for the case manager leading to burnout or turnover.

Kane, R. A. Case management: ethical pitfalls on the road to high-quality managed care. *Quality Review Bulletin* 14(5):161–68, 1988.

> Kane points out that case management is confronted with a dual perspective: advocacy versus utilization and cost containment. An advocacy perspective, embedded in the historical traditions of social work and public health nursing, calls for partisan efforts to assist people experiencing health problems and crises to obtain and utilize whatever resources they need to meet their needs or perhaps preferences. An alternative perspective is that case management must husband services and perhaps even ration them to those individuals who are in most need. Kane believes that these alternative perspectives create serious ethical pitfalls. Cost containment may place constraints on advocacy. An advocacy perspective raises the issue of whether people can optimize their preferences in light of scarce resources. Readers will want to review this article in

order to understand how to frame the purpose of a case management program.

The Issue of Professional Discipline and Training

Applebaum, R. A., and Wilson, N. L. Training needs for providing case management for the long-term care client: lessons from the National Channeling Demonstration. *The Gerontologist* 28(2):172–76, 1988.

This paper documents the training needs of case managers involved in long-term care identified through a national demonstration project. Three major categories of training needs were identified: a need to understand the client (for example, health and disability issues, mental health concerns, and morbidity and mortality factors); a need to understand the environment (for example, understanding service providers, eligibility, interdisciplinary practice, and service costs); and a need to become proficient in the use of case management techniques. The project findings call for a need to train case managers in areas outside of their discipline because of biases reinforced by preservice education. Case managers who did not accept a broad role definition tended to become frustrated with long-term care work. Those social workers who emphasized counseling and those nurses who emphasized hands-on medical care tended to drop out of the project at a rate higher than those professionals who assumed more flexibility in their roles.

Hurley, R. E. Toward a behavioral model of the physician as case manager. *Social Science and Medicine* 23(1):75–82, 1986.

This paper discusses the pivotal role that physicians hold in relationship to resource consumption decisions and, therefore, the primary care physician serves a crucial role in case management that goes beyond traditional clinical responsibilities of the physician. Physician case management involves the function of a specific physician as the "point of entry" into the health care system for a patient. The model formulated by Hurley involves role choices involving healer, coordinator, expert, and rationer. This functional set is created through the intersection of service orientation (patient versus self-interest) and skills orientation (clinical versus managerial) that the physician can manipulate in order to create case management practice. An emphasis placed on coordination, for example, integrates a focus on patient needs that are driven by managerial concerns. This paper illustrates the variety of decisions that a discipline can make to formulate different case management role packages. It also highlights and illustrates the involvement of primary care physicians in health care case management.

Johnson, P. J., and Rubin, A. Case management in mental health: a social work domain? *Social Work* 28(1):49–55, 1983.

> This paper represents an early argument about who should undertake case management — an issue that expresses itself in contemporary programs and program development efforts. Johnson and Rubin argue that case management lacks clarity in its conceptualization and even in its basic definitions but that there is a similarity and complementarity of social work roles and case management functions in responding to the needs of people with serious mental illness. This similarity and complementarity is buttressed within the context of social work education, professional commitments, and sequencing of professional levels. But, Johnson and Rubin emphasize that practicing social workers did not express preferences for engaging in these roles. The authors note that social workers may be "indifferent" to the assumption of case management roles and responsibilities.

The Issue of Case Management Purpose

Anthony, W. A., Cohen, M., Farkas, M., and Cohen, B. F. Case management — more than a response to a dysfunctional system. *Community Mental Health Journal* 24(3):219–28, 1988.

> The authors assert that case management was founded as a response to dysfunctional service delivery systems characterized by fragmentation and uncoordination. However, the authors maintain that case management will be needed no matter how well a system functions since effective case management responds to the goals of consumers rather than to the needs of the system. Case management is seen in the context of this paper as a process of consumer support in which clients are assisted in negotiating for the services and supports they want for themselves. Thus, case management is a form of advocacy and focuses on addressing client self-defined goals and pressing the system for service improvements. The ultimate purpose of case management is to humanize an administratively-driven system by offering consumers a relationship with a dedicated advocate.

Dixon, T. P., Goll, S., and Stanton, K. M. Case management issues and practices in head injury rehabilitation. *Rehabilitation Counseling Bulletin* 31:325–43, 1988.

> This paper is very relevant in light of the growing issue of cost containment, service relevance, and broad-based service needs created by people who have experienced traumatic head injury. The authors note that

the "sheer magnitude of the numbers of head injury survivors, as well as the complexity of disability and subsequent recovery patterns" have created substantial growth in models, programs, and services dedicated to head injury rehabilitation. The authors assert that the purpose of head injury case management is to assure the quality of head injury rehabilitation services and to serve as a "cost–benefit guide" through complex service systems characterized by multiple models and levels of care. This approach to case management has been complemented by a gradual movement of the head injury service system away from "more is better" to a decision-based approach that incorporates a data-driven outcome framework that is measurable and functional. Service complexity, the high costs and length of care, and the need to measure outcome rather than effort has created a need for head injury case management to form alliances among family members, consumers, and the funders of care. The purpose of these alliances is to create accountability so that effective cost–benefit decisions are formulated in a manner that is responsive to the needs of consumers.

Additional Books of Interest

Measuring Outcomes in Ambulatory Care
by Dale S. Benson, M.D.

This book presents a practical approach to measuring effectiveness in the episodic environment of ambulatory care. Explained is a detailed, step-by-step process for developing effective outcome indicators, classified into four categories — disease specific, general health, patient performance, and patient satisfaction. This approach is designed for all types of ambulatory care in all kinds of settings.

Catalog no. E99-169106 (must be included when ordering)
1992. 192 pages, 6 appendixes, 31 figures and tables.
$49.95 (AHA members, $39.95)

Hospital Home Care: Strategic Management for Integrated Care Delivery
edited by Dan Lerman, M.H.S.A., Lerman & Company, Memphis and Chicago; and Eric B. Linne, J.D., of the AHA Division of Ambulatory Care

With chapters by some of the foremost authorities in the hospital home care field, *Hospital Home Care: Strategic Management for Integrated Care Delivery* will provide hospital administrators and home care managers with timely, critical information on planning and operating home care programs. This book presents the best way to analyze market opportunities in the community, and contains many of the essential "how-tos" in starting and operating a variety of hospital home care service lines.

Catalog no. E99-079200 (must be included when ordering)
1993. 328 pages, 64 figures, 26 tables.
$60.00 (AHA members, $48.00)

To order, call TOLL FREE
1-800-AHA-2626